HANDBOOK OF
Retinal Screening
in Diabetes

HANDBOOK OF
Retinal Screening in Diabetes

ROY TAYLOR

Department of Diabetes and Metabolism
The Medical School, University of Newcastle upon Tyne
and Newcastle Diabetes Centre

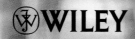WILEY

Other Wiley Editorial Offices

John Wiley & Sons Inc., 111 River Street, Hoboken, NJ 07030, USA

Jossey-Bass, 989 Market Street, San Francisco, CA 94103-1741, USA

Wiley-VCH Verlag GmbH, Boschstr. 12, D-69469 Weinheim, Germany

John Wiley & Sons Australia Ltd, 33 Park Road, Milton, Queensland 4064, Australia

John Wiley & Sons (Asia) Pte Ltd, 2 Clementi Loop #02-01, Jin Xing Distripark, Singapore
129809

John Wiley & Sons Canada Ltd, 22 Worcester Road, Etobicoke, Ontario, Canada M9W 1L1

Wiley also publishes its books in a variety of electronic formats. Some content that appears in
print may not be available in electronic books.

Library of Congress Cataloging-in-Publication Data

Taylor, Roy, 1952–
   Handbook of retinal screening in diabetes / Roy Taylor.
      p. ; cm.
   Includes bibliographical references.
   ISBN-13: 978-0-470-02882-7 (alk. paper)
   ISBN-10: 0-470-02882-3 (alk. paper)
   1. Diabetic retinopathy—Diagnosis—Handbooks, manuals, etc.   I. Title.
   [DNLM: 1. Diabetic Retinopathy—diagnosis—Handbooks. WK 39
   T245h 2006]
   RE661.D5T35 2006
   617.7′3—dc22
2006001394

British Library Cataloguing in Publication Data

A catalogue record for this book is available from the British Library

ISBN-13 0-978-0-470-02882-7
ISBN-10 0-470-02882-3

Typeset in 10.5/13 pt Sabon
Printed in Spain by Grafos, Barcelona
This book is printed on acid-free paper responsibly manufactured from sustainable forestry in
which at least two trees are planted for each one used for paper production.

Contents

Preface

This book has been written mainly for retinal screeners, but should be of interest to others including optometrists, medical students, nurses, diabetologists and ophthalmologists. It describes diabetes from the perspective of the patient, acknowledging the day to day difficulties which are often unknown to those who do not themselves have diabetes. The book also covers the basic anatomy of the eye, visual function and the practicalities of screening individuals and populations. However, the most important chapters describe retinal images to allow acquisition of the vital skill of recognizing different degrees of severity of retinopathy.

Retinal screening is part of diabetes care, and retinal screeners play a vital role in the diabetes care team which delivers the service to individuals with diabetes. Although the book is intended primarily as a practical handbook, it should be useful for those preparing to take the new UK National Diploma in diabetes retinal screening.

All images were taken using Canon CR-6 cameras with either JVC or Canon D60 digital imagers. The images in this book have all been taken during routine screening in busy sessions. Experts on eyes or photographs may feel that their technical quality is not optimal. However, this is a book about practical screening in diabetes and deals with the reality of image interpretation in day to day work. It is not a textbook of ophthalmology. The level of resolution obtained is easily sufficient to detect treatable retinopathy and prevent diabetes blindness. Indeed, the major fall in rates of blindness in Newcastle upon Tyne was achieved using lower resolution Polaroid retinal photographs.

The self-assessment chapter has been organized so that you may test yourself after each chapter. The retinal images are also obtainable from the web, and the website can be used as a further self-assessment tool.

This book could not have been put together without the expert input of the Newcastle retinal screening team – Denise Young, Deborah Batey, Maureen Shotton, Diane Mitchie and Dianne Mitchell. I am most grateful to each of them, and this book is an attempt to clone them. Dr C.S. Arun helped to identify representative images and Dr Ayad Al-Bermani, Medical Ophthalmologist, proof read the book. Photographs were taken by Jodie Batey and line drawings were created by James Corris. My knowledge about diabetic retinopathy has been acquired by close and much appreciated collaboration over many years with Mr Kevin Stannard, Consultant Ophthalmologist.

Roy Taylor

How to Use This Book

The first five chapters are intended to be self-contained – so that they can be read or not depending upon the needs of the reader. A summary of important information is provided as a Fact File at the end of each of these chapters. Self-assessment questions for each chapter are given in Chapter 13.

When examining the images in Chapters 6 to 11 it is essential to use a bright light such as a desk lamp or be close to a bright reading lamp. Diffuse fluorescent lighting is particularly poor for seeing fine retinal details. However, to allow the viewing of images as they would be seen during screening – full size upon a screen – a website has been created for the use of readers of this book. It can be found at www.servier.co.uk/retinalimagebank. The images may be viewed and then the descriptive text may be read to allow consideration of all the features.

The chapter on background information will introduce to people new to clinical diabetes or retinal screening the general knowledge which will benefit their patients. Updated information will be displayed at www.servier.co.uk/retinalimagebank as necessary, so check this website from time to time.

1

Type 1 Diabetes

What causes type 1 diabetes?

Diabetes is a disorder in which blood glucose levels are high. In normal health, blood glucose levels are precisely controlled by the hormone insulin. This is made by the beta cells in the pancreas gland, an organ behind the stomach. Minute to minute control of insulin production by the beta cells normally keeps blood glucose levels constant. After a meal, the rate of insulin production rises sharply.

Type 1 diabetes is the result of destruction of the beta cells in the pancreas. This is most often caused by the body's defence mechanisms attacking the cells as though they were invaders (an 'autoimmune' process). The process of beta cell destruction happens over a period of many months, but symptoms can start very suddenly once the number of functioning beta cells falls to a critical level.

Who gets type 1 diabetes?

Type 1 diabetes used to be called juvenile onset diabetes. It can occur any time from early childhood into late adult life, but starts most commonly in early adolescence. The condition is slightly more likely to occur if family members have type 1 diabetes, but many people have no such family history.

Approximately 0.2 per cent of children of school age have type 1 diabetes in the UK. In the population as a whole it affects around 0.3 per cent.

Handbook of Retinal Screening in Diabetes, Roy Taylor
© 2006 John Wiley & Sons, Ltd

How does it present?

The main symptoms come on over a period of weeks and are:

- thirst
- passing large amounts of urine
- weight loss
- tiredness
- skin infections, especially thrush.

There will be glucose (sugar) present in the urine. Also, ketones are likely to be present in the urine. Ketones are the by-product of fat breakdown and are normal in trace amounts for anyone during fasting. However, excessive amounts of ketones are only present in urine when lack of insulin allows fat to break down excessively.

Essentials of management

Insulin

Insulin must be replaced to maintain life. As the insulin molecule is a peptide (a small protein), it would be broken down in the stomach if swallowed – just like any protein food. Insulin has to be injected into the fat layer under the skin. This may be done using a disposable syringe with insulin drawn from a vial, or by using a pen injector (Figure 1.1). Insulin is usually advised to be injected through the skin into the fatty tissue of the abdomen, the upper thighs or hips.

There are two basic types of insulin regime. A combined injection of short-acting insulin and intermediate acting insulin may be given before breakfast and before the evening meal (Figure 1.2). This has the advantage of simplicity, but the disadvantage that meals have to be eaten at fairly fixed times and in fairly fixed quantities.

The second regime tries to mimic the normal situation, with a low background of insulin being provided by a single daily injection of longer-acting insulin, together with the use of very short-acting insulin taken at a time when it is convenient to eat a meal, and in an amount corresponding to the size of that meal. Although this may involve three or more injections per day of very short-acting insulin, these can be given using a convenient pen device.

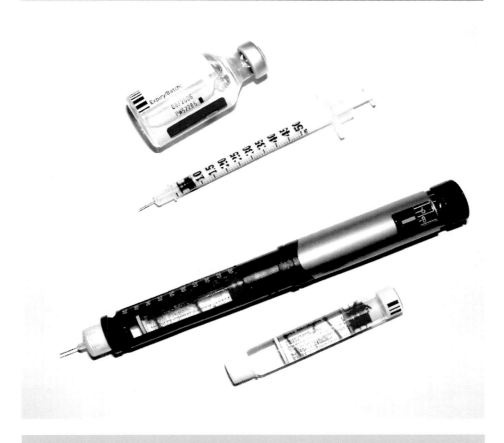

Figure 1.1 Insulin pens contain a 3 ml cartridge of insulin and are convenient to use as the required dose can rapidly be set and then injected; This avoids having to draw up a dose of insulin into a syringe from a vial

The names of some of the commonly used insulins are listed in Table 1.1.

Food

People with diabetes can eat normally, with a few modifications. Overall, the pattern of eating advised is merely that of a healthy lifestyle – not too much sugar,

Normal pattern in non-diabetic people

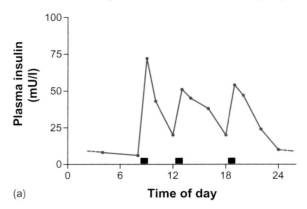

(a)

Daily insulin levels on twice daily short- and longer-acting insulin

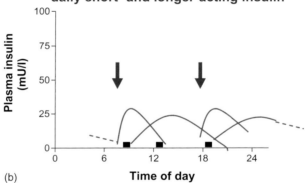

(b)

Daily insulin levels on basal /bolus insulin regime

(c)

Table 1.1 Commonly used insulins and their time of action; the names in each box refer to similar insulins made by different manufacturers

Insulin	Time of action	Use
Humalog® Novorapid®	0 min–2 hours *Very short*	As meal boluses (single doses)
Actrapid® Humulin S®	15 min–6 hours *Short*	1. As part of a twice daily short- and intermediate-acting insulin regime 2. As meal boluses with evening intermediate-acting insulin
Humulin I® Insulatard®	1–14 hours *Intermediate*	1. As part of a twice daily short- and intermediate-acting insulin regime 2. As overnight insulin (used with short-acting insulin to cover meals)
Lantus®	1–24 hours *Long*	As basal insulin (used with boluses of very short-acting insulin to cover meals)

avoid fatty foods, and plenty fruit and vegetables. Carbohydrate foods such as bread, pasta, potatoes and biscuits need to be considered in determining what dose of insulin is required. Since the 1930s carbohydrate has been 'counted' as 10 g exchanges. For instance, an apple, a small potato or a digestive biscuit each can be counted as a 10 g exchange of carbohydrate. A person with diabetes is trained to assess how many carbohydrate exchanges would be in a meal.

Figure 1.2 (a) Insulin levels normally increase sharply after meals, and fall back towards a low baseline afterwards; the black boxes show the meal times. (b) This shows in a diagrammatic form what happens when a dose of short-acting insulin and a dose of longer-acting insulin are injected before breakfast and before the evening meal. This insulin regime is simple, but does mean that meals have to be eaten at predictable times. (c) This shows similar information when a basal (very long-acting) insulin is injected before bed to provide a low background of insulin to mimic the normal situation. Doses of very short-acting insulin are given before meals, and there is flexibility both in the timing and size of meals

Hypoglycaemia

This word merely means 'low blood glucose' and is usually shortened to 'hypo'. Hypos occur when the balance of injected insulin and food eaten is not correct. If, for instance, only a small meal had been taken despite a dose of insulin appropriate for a larger meal having already been injected, then the insulin would have too great an effect upon blood glucose and the level will fall (Figure 1.3).

A hypo causes sweating, shakiness, a feeling of great hunger and eventually muddled thinking. If it is not treated by eating some sugary food, the muddled thinking will get worse, and eventually consciousness will be lost. There is a great risk that a person may be assumed to have drunk too much alcohol because of the uncoordinated movements and confusion.

Especially after many years of type 1 diabetes, awareness of the early symptoms of hypos becomes blunted. There is then a risk of loss of consciousness without warning. The treatment of hypoglycaemia is administration of any sugary drink. A hypoglycaemic person may be uncooperative. Treatment from a doctor or paramedic would involve intravenous administration of glucose, or subcutaneous injection of glucagon. Glucagon is a hormone which has an opposite effect to that of insulin and causes the liver to produce glucose.

Ketoacidosis

If a person with type 1 diabetes did not take insulin, glucose could not be used by the body and fat (the main alternative fuel) would be mobilized excessively. High levels of ketones would be present in the blood and urine. As ketones are weak acids, the blood becomes slightly acidic. Nausea and then vomiting occurs. Once vomiting starts the condition is likely to be fatal within one to two days unless treated.

Anyone with type 1 diabetes who is ill is advised to test their blood glucose frequently and also to test their urine for ketones. The insulin dose always needs to be increased during illness, even if no food is eaten (because the body becomes resistant to ordinary levels of insulin). It is vital that expert medical help is obtained. Hospital admission is necessary for established ketoacidosis.

Living with type 1 diabetes

Few people who do not have type 1 diabetes actually appreciate the difficulty of living with a condition which requires attention every time the person wishes to eat or exercise.

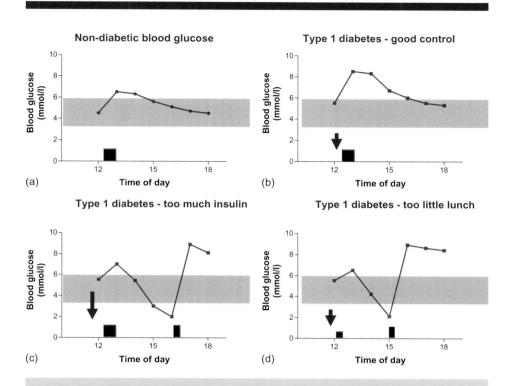

Figure 1.3 (a) In non-diabetic people, blood glucose levels rise after eating, but the rise is limited by the normal insulin response and smooth control is achieved whatever the size of the meal. In all the graphs the meal size is represented by the black boxes and the normal pre-meal range of glucose is shown by the shaded area. (b) In well controlled type 1 diabetes the rise in blood glucose after eating is likely to be greater than normal, but if the insulin dose (represented by the arrow) matches the meal size then control will be achieved. (c) If too great a dose of insulin was given the rise after the meal would be smaller and blood glucose levels will fall below the normal range. Symptoms of hypo would draw attention to the need for extra food, and blood glucose levels tend to overshoot. (d) If only a small lunch was taken with a dose of insulin of usual size then blood glucose levels will rise little before the insulin causes a fall. Again, symptoms of hypo would occur, extra food would be taken and blood glucose levels will overshoot

To maintain the fine balance between blood glucose levels that are too high or too low requires detailed understanding of diabetes as well as hour to hour effort every single day. Adjusting insulin regimes to fit with work patterns, including shift work, is not always straightforward. In practice, individuals adopt habits which lead to average blood glucose levels which reflect a compromise that they themselves can tolerate. These are often higher than might be ideal, but considerable empathy and insight into individual circumstances is required before it can be said that control 'must' be better. Most other people in the diabetes team do not need to take diabetes home with them.

During any minor illness the need for insulin rises and major adjustments are needed to keep control.

In order to hold a driving licence people with diabetes have to be able to recognize the early symptoms of hypoglycaemia, and have to obey the driving rules:

- test blood glucose before driving;
- always keep glucose tablets or sweets in the car;
- plan longer journeys to ensure appropriate stops for snacks.

Blood glucose testing

It is only possible to 'know' one's own blood glucose level if it is either very high or very low. For this reason it is important for people with diabetes to be able to test their blood glucose level. By using a finger pricking device, a tiny drop of blood can be obtained. This is placed on a disposable strip connected to a meter (Figure 1.4).

The level of glucose in blood is measured in millimoles per litre (mmol/l). The non-diabetic fasting range for blood glucose is 3.5 to 5.5 mmol/l. In type 1 diabetes blood glucose levels would ideally be between 4 and 7 mmol/l before meals, but in practice much higher numbers may be observed. For each individual, a target range will have been agreed. In very long-standing type 1 diabetes blood glucose levels may vary unpredictably and it may be necessary to aim for higher numbers in order to avoid very frequent hypos.

Complications

High blood glucose levels for many years can damage the smallest blood vessels – capillaries. The particular tissues which are most affected by this process are the retina, nerves and kidney. These complications are known as 'microvascular' complications. The number of people with such complications increases as the duration of type 1 diabetes increases (see Figure 4.2).

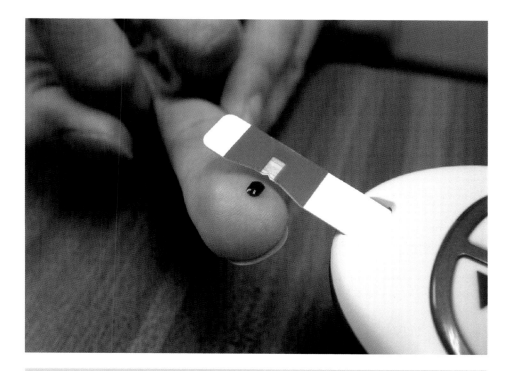

Figure 1.4 To test blood glucose, a short needle is used to prick the finger and the drop of blood is placed on the test strip; the strip is connected to a small meter which gives a read-out of the result within seconds

Large blood vessels are also affected by high blood glucose levels. These 'macrovascular' complications include premature heart attacks, strokes and poor circulation to the feet. Diabetes causes fat to be deposited in the arterial walls, accelerating atherosclerosis (hardening of the arteries).

The risk of developing these long-term complications of diabetes is directly related to how well the diabetes is controlled. It is possible to assess this by a single blood test which indicates the average blood glucose levels over a period of two months. This is possible as glucose becomes attached to the pigment in red blood cells (haemoglobin). The amount of glucose attached to haemoglobin is measured in the test as 'HbA1c'. In non-diabetic people, the normal amount of glucose in the blood causes the level of HbA1c to be up to 6.0 per cent. A very well motivated person with type 1 diabetes may be able to achieve an HbA1c of 7.5 per cent or less. Some people can only manage to achieve HbA1c levels of over 12 per cent. A major study carried out in the US demonstrated very clearly the relationship between HbA1c and the chance of developing complications. In general, the higher the HbA1c, the higher the risk of developing complications.

A further important factor is that of blood pressure. In diabetes, the higher the blood pressure, the faster complications will develop. Very tight control of blood pressure has been shown to have a greater effect than very tight control of blood glucose in slowing the rate of progression of complications. Although this may seem surprising at first, it has to be seen as a series of stages:

1. high blood glucose damages the capillaries and arteries

2. high blood pressure will cause the damaged capillaries to leak or burst

3. reversal of high blood pressure will have an immediate effect upon the well-being of blood vessels

4. reversal of high blood glucose will just slow further damage

However, it has to be recognized that some people appear to be less susceptible to complications than others. Other unknown factors determine the risk of complications for any one individual.

History

The word 'diabetes' comes from the Greek word for a siphon. This illustrates very clearly the main symptoms of type 1 diabetes – constant excessive drinking and passing of urine. The first written reference to diabetes dates back to 1500 BC. In 1889 Oscar Minkowski discovered that removal of the pancreas caused diabetes in animals. In 1921 Banting, Best, Collip and McLeod discovered a method of purifying insulin extracted from animals' pancreases. The first patient to be treated with insulin received a dose in January 1922. Previously type 1 diabetes was more rapidly fatal then most cancers, and insulin was hailed as a cure for diabetes. However, by the 1930s it was clear that long-term complications became very troublesome.

Fact file

- Type 1 diabetes is caused by destruction of the beta cells of the pancreas.

- The problems of type 1 diabetes are primarily due to failure to produce insulin.

- Treatment consists of injecting insulin in a pattern to balance carbohydrate food.

- Too much insulin, too little food or unaccustomed physical activity causes hypoglycaemia (hypo).

- Hypos cause some or all of: sweating, shakiness, incoordination, aggressive behaviour and eventually unconsciousness.

- Hypos are treated by giving anything containing sugar.

- Illness in type 1 diabetes may cause ketoacidosis and need for hospital admission.

- HbA1c is a measure of average blood glucose over about 2 months.

- Microvascular complications include damage to the retina, nerves and kidney.

- Macrovascular complications include premature heart attack, strokes and poor circulation.

- The rate of development of complications can be slowed by tight control of blood pressure and blood glucose.

Further reading

1. http://www.diabetes.org.uk/home.htm
2. Day, J.L. (2002) *Living With Diabetes: The Diabetes UK Guide for those Treated with Insulin*, John Wiley & Sons, Ltd, Cluchester.
3. http://diabetes.niddk.nih.gov/dm/pubs/control/

2
Type 2 Diabetes

What causes type 2 diabetes?

Type 2 diabetes is the result of two processes. First, the insulin-producing beta cells in the pancreas become less able to make insulin in response to eating. The exact cause of this is not clear, but it is estimated that the process has been underway for approximately 10 years before the condition is diagnosed. Secondly, the tissues of the body that respond to insulin – largely muscle and the liver – are resistant to insulin. In other words, even though reasonable levels of insulin may be present the tissues do not respond to it.

It is clear that being overweight plays a role in causing type 2 diabetes. In societies where obesity is rare, type 2 diabetes is also rare. If a person is overweight and they have a tendency to diabetes, the condition will develop decades before it would do if body weight was normal. When such societies become 'Westernised' with less daily physical exercise and more food, obesity rates rise and diabetes becomes common. This explains the current epidemic rise in numbers of people with diabetes in Europe and North America.

Who gets type 2 diabetes?

Type 2 diabetes used to be called maturity onset diabetes (or non-insulin dependent diabetes). It is usually diagnosed after the age of 30 years but is commonest in older people. Occasionally it now occurs in adolescents,

Handbook of Retinal Screening in Diabetes, Roy Taylor
© 2006 John Wiley & Sons, Ltd

usually associated with gross obesity. One third of people presenting with type 2 diabetes have a family history of the condition affecting parents or sisters and brothers.

It affects approximately 3 per cent of the UK population as a whole. Some subgroups are particularly susceptible, and the prevalence in Asian people living in the UK is approximately 10 per cent.

How does it present?

Type 2 diabetes is often diagnosed at a routine check up with glucose (sugar) being found in a urine sample. It can be present without causing any symptoms for years. However, left untreated it will cause some or all of the following symptoms:

- skin infections, especially thrush
- urinary infections
- tiredness
- thirst
- passing large amounts of urine

Management

It is important to realize that type 2 diabetes is constantly progressing in each individual. If diagnosed early, diet alone can achieve good control. However, within months or years tablet treatment will usually become necessary. Some years later, insulin treatment will be needed. Once diabetes is established, this rate of progress cannot be affected by diet, tablets or insulin even though blood glucose levels will be improved by treatment.

Eating

People with diabetes can eat normally, with modifications. Note that the word 'diet' is best avoided as 'diets' are regarded as those things read about in magazines and never followed for more than a week. Most published diets reflect the need to entertain rather than to convey sensible information. Overall, the pattern of eating advised for a person with type 2 diabetes is merely that of a healthy lifestyle – not too much sugar, few fatty foods, and plenty of fruit and vegetables.

For all of us most energy is obtained from carbohydrate and fat. In order to take in enough food energy for day to day life, carbohydrate foods such as bread, pasta and potatoes need to be taken in adequate amounts and too much fat avoided. In practice this means no fried foods, no prepared meals and avoiding too much red meat and dairy produce. The change in eating pattern has to be adopted by the whole family to be sustainable for one person. There are health benefits for all in this approach.

Calorie restriction is important for all people with type 2 diabetes. This restriction has to be consistent and of long duration to make an impact on body weight. Temporary diets are of no value. Beer and wine contain calories (1 pint of beer averages 200 calories; 1 glass of wine averages 70 calories) and avoiding excessive alcohol consumption must be considered as part of calorie restriction. Alcohol itself in moderation has no adverse consequences in type 2 diabetes.

Physical activity

People are encouraged to walk instead of using car or bus, to take the stairs not the lift and if possible to undertake recreational activity.

It is the everyday, long-term energy expenditure which matters. Body weight is the long-term result of two processes: how much food energy is taken in and how much energy is expended. If the body is left with a surplus, this is stored in the form of fat. Going to a gym on a few occasions will achieve little in terms of weight loss, whereas merely walking for 20 minutes per day will achieve 2.5 kg (5.5 pounds) weight loss over a year. It is for this reason that government action on a transport policy (less car use, more walking, cycling and use of public transport) would achieve far more in terms of preventing obesity than campaigns providing dietary advice.

There are two reasons for advising physical activity. Firstly, it will help with energy balance. People gain weight if they eat more calories than they burn in everyday life. Secondly, people with type 2 diabetes are especially susceptible to heart attacks and strokes, and regular physical exercise helps to minimize this risk.

Tablets

When adjustment of eating patterns fails to achieve good blood glucose control despite an individual's best efforts then tablet treatment will be advised. One major factor for the success of tablets is that they must be taken regularly. You know that last time you had to take a course of antibiotics you probably missed several doses, even though this was only for a few days. When tablets are prescribed for long-term conditions, establishing the daily (or twice daily) habit is vital, using whatever cues are appropriate. Open discussion of this problem between patient and doctor (or nurse) can be helpful.

There are three types of tablet in use at the present time which may be used singly or in double or triple combination.

Metformin

This tablet has been in use since the 1950s. It acts on the liver to decrease production of glucose. It has the side effect of causing diarrhoea especially when first started. For this reason it is started at a low dose then increased.

Sulphonylureas

This group of medicines acts by stimulating insulin production by the beta cells of the pancreas. They have the potential side effect of pushing the blood glucose level too low, especially if the person stops eating for any reason. Hypos can be caused, just as in the case of insulin treatment.

Glitazones

Pioglitazone and rosiglitazone are relatively new drugs which increase the body's sensitivity to insulin. Their main side effect is that they can cause fluid retention and swollen ankles in susceptible people. Some new evidence suggests that they may be able to slow the rate of deterioration towards needing insulin therapy although this needs to be proved further.

Other tablets

In type 2 diabetes there are three main quantities to control: blood glucose, blood pressure and blood lipids. For any one individual, up to three tablets may be taken for blood glucose control, up to five for blood pressure control and up to two for blood lipid control. In addition, other tablets are used commonly. Table 2.1 lists some of the frequently used tablets. This is not an exhausive list, but indicates the range and number of tablets which may be advised. Several trade names may be in use for any one drug, and a representative one is listed. (Do not try to learn this table).

Insulin

Insulin may be injected by syringe or pen device if needed. Many people with type 2 diabetes may be given twice daily longer-acting insulin, relying on the pancreas to help after meals. It is now becoming commoner for both tablets and insulin to be used in combination. The main side effect of insulin therapy is hypoglycaemia (see Chapter 1).

Living with type 2 diabetes

The main challenge for people with type 2 diabetes is to change the lifestyle which allowed the condition to develop in the first place. Changing the habits of a lifetime is not easy, and individuals differ in how successful they are in the long term.

Blood glucose and urine testing

Glucose spills over into the urine when levels in the blood are too high (around 11 mmol/l). Urine testing can be useful as a general check that control is not deteriorating. For exact information on blood glucose levels, direct measurement is necessary. By using a finger pricking device, a tiny drop of blood is placed on a disposable strip connected to a meter (Figure 1.4).

The non-diabetic fasting range for blood glucose is 3.5 to 5.5 mmol/l. In type 2 diabetes, advised blood glucose levels depend upon the clinical aims of treatment. These differ between, say, a middle-aged active person who is otherwise fit and a frail older person. For tightest control blood glucose would ideally be between 4 and 7 mmol/l before meals. For each individual, a target range will have been agreed.

Complications

High blood glucose levels for many years can damage the smallest blood vessels – just as in type 1 diabetes. The complications of high blood glucose

Table 2.1   Commonly used tablets for people with type 2 diabetes

Name	Trade name	Group	Main action
Glucose control			
Gliclazide	Diamicron Diamicron MR	Sulphonylurea	Increases insulin secretion
Glibenclamide	Euglucon	Sulphonylurea	Increases insulin secretion
Repaglinide	Novonorm	Benzoic acid derivative	Increases insulin secretion
Nateglinide	Starlix	Nateglinide	Increases insulin secretion
Metformin	Glucophage Glucophage SR	Biguanide	Increases insulin action
Pioglitazone	Actos	Thiazolidinedione	Increases insulin action
Rosiglitazone	Avandia	Thiazolidinedione	Increases insulin action
Blood pressure			
Lisinopril	Carace/Zestril	ACE inhibitor	Inhibits renin system
Perindopril	Coversyl	ACE inhibitor	Inhibits renin system
Indapamide	Natrilix	Diuretic	Promotes sodium excretion
Bendrofluazide	Aprinox	Diuretic	Promotes sodium excretion
Nifedipine	Adalat	Calcium channel blocker	Dilates arteries
Amlodipine	Istin	Calcium channel blocker	Dilates arteries
Atenolol	Tenormin	Beta blocker	Decreases adrenaline effect
Doxazosin	Cardura	Alpha blocker	Decreases adrenaline effect
Irbesartan	Aprovel	Angiotensin II antagonist	Inhibits renin system
Candesartan	Amias	Angiotensin II antagonist	Inhibits renin system
Lipids			
Simvastatin	Zocor	Statin	Inhibits cholesterol synthesis
Atorvastatin	Lipitor	Statin	Inhibits cholesterol synthesis
Ezetimibe	Ezetrol	Absorption inhibitor	Inhibits cholesterol absorption
Bezafibrate	Bezalip	Fibric acid	Lowers triglyceride
Fenofibrate	Lipantil	Fibric acid	Lowers triglyceride
Omega 3	Omacor	Omega 3 fatty ester	Lowers triglyceride
Anti-thrombotic			
Aspirin	Aspirin	Anti-platelet agent	Inhibits platelets clumping
Clopidogrel	Plavix	Anti-platelet agent	Inhibits platelets clumping
Anti-obesity			
Orlistat	Zenical	Intestinal lipase inhibitor	Inhibits fat absorption

levels are the same whatever the cause of the diabetes (see Chapter 1). The time course of complications differs from that in type 1 diabetes. The major difference is that serious complications may already be present at the time of diagnosis of type 2 diabetes. Indeed, they may cause the condition to be diagnosed. The effect of duration upon the presence of retinopathy is shown in Figure 2.1 (a).

Large blood vessels are affected by high blood glucose levels especially in type 2 diabetes. These macrovascular complications include premature heart attacks, strokes and poor circulation to the feet (Figure 2.1(b)).

As in type 1 diabetes, the rate of progression of long-term complications is directly related to how well the diabetes is controlled. The largest and

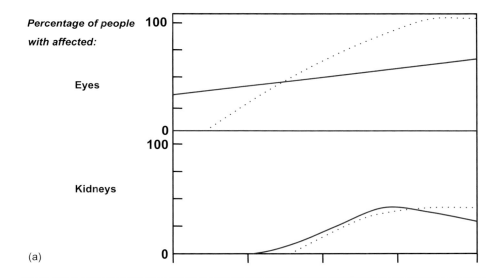

(a)

Figure 2.1 (a)   The rate of increase in the percentage of people affected by complications is shown as the duration of diabetes increases. The lines are very different for each type of diabetes. At the time of diagnosis of type 2 diabetes approximately 35 per cent of people already have some degree of diabetic retinopathy. This increases steadily over the subsequent years. In type 1 diabetes, retinopathy typically does not develop for several years. Diabetic kidney disease tends to be a late complication in both types of diabetes, but is seen earlier in type 2 diabetes. Bear in mind that the lines show only the average, and there is wide variation between individuals. (Type 1 dotted line, type 2 solid line)

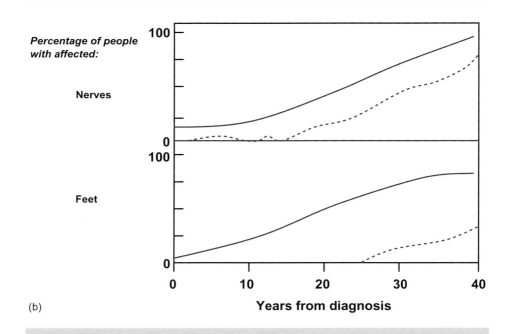

(b)

Figure 2.1 (b) In type 2 diabetes, over 10 per cent of people already have nerve damage at diagnosis, and there is a steady rise such that most people are affected after 40 years of diabetes. In type 1 diabetes, nerve damage can be intermittent, but typically the prevalence rises steadily after around 15 years of diabetes. Foot problems are common in type 2 diabetes, but are seen only in the later stages of type 1 diabetes (type 1 dotted line, type 2 solid line)

longest randomized, prospective study ever conducted was the UK Prospective Diabetes Study (UKPDS). This showed that doing all possible to improve blood glucose control decreased eye, nerve and kidney problems by about 25 per cent. It also suggested that heart attacks and strokes were decreased by about 15 per cent in the well controlled group.

The UKPDS showed for the first time that very active treatment of blood pressure slowed down the development of eye, nerve, kidney and heart complications (Figure 4.6). As tight control of blood pressure caused a 37 per cent decrease in microvascular problems and a 44 per cent decrease in the risk of a stroke, it is even more effective to treat high blood pressure than to decrease blood glucose levels. In practice, of course, both are important aims of treatment.

However, it has to be recognized that some people appear to be less susceptible to complications than others. Other unknown factors determine the risk of complications for any one individual. A further important factor is that of blood pressure. In diabetes, the higher the blood pressure, the faster complications will develop.

History

Type 2 diabetes was not recognized as a completely distinct condition from type 1 diabetes until the mid 1930s. This was the work of Harold Himsworth, a UK physician.

However, a French physician called Bouchardet noticed that during the siege of Paris in 1870 most of his patients with diabetes became better controlled. Glucose disappeared from their urine. It is now clear that this was the effect of enforced calorie restriction on people with type 2 diabetes.

The effect of lifestyle and obesity is made clear by another observation. When the famous American diabetologist Elliot Joslin visited the Pima Indians in Arizona in the 1890s, he commented that it was remarkable that the tribe had no people with diabetes. At that time the Pimas were subsistence farmers. A century later, displaced from their lands, unemployed and receiving government food aid, obesity is common and 40 per cent of the Pima Indians have diabetes. Populations who have been genetically selected over centuries for survival in conditions of scarce food seem to be especially susceptible to the effects of inactivity and overeating.

Further reading

1. http://www.diabetes.org.uk/home.htm
2. Day, J.L. (2001) *Living with Diabetes: the Diabetes UK Guide for those Treated with Diet and Tablets*, John Wiley & Sons, Ltd, Cluchester.
3. Ganz, M. (ed) (2005) *Prevention of Type 2 Diabetes*, John Wiley & Sons, Ltd, Cluchester.

Fact file

- Age of onset is usually over 40 years, but this is falling.

- Type 2 diabetes is caused by a partial failure of insulin secretion coupled with a poor response to insulin.

- The defect in insulin secretion gradually worsens over years.

- Treatment consists of a low sugar, low fat pattern of eating at first.

- When control cannot be obtained by adjusting eating, tablet treatment is added.

- When tablets cannot achieve good control, insulin treatment becomes necessary.

- HbA1c is a measure of average blood glucose over about 2 months.

- Microvascular complications include damage to the retina, nerves and kidney.

- Macrovascular complications include premature heart attack, strokes and poor circulation.

- Good control of blood glucose slows the rate of progression of complications.

- Good control of blood pressure has a greater effect in slowing the rate of progression of complications.

3

The Eye in Diabetes

Structure of the normal eye

The eye is a specialized organ which detects light. It is essentially a globe with a window (Figure 3.1). Light passes through the cornea and is detected by the retina which lines the inside of the globe. Nerve fibres run across the retina and carry information to the brain in the optic nerve.

Figure 3.2 shows the eye as it appears in everyday life. Protection for the delicate cornea is provided by the upper and lower eyelids. The coloured iris acts as a regulator, causing the pupil to be small in bright light (shutting out too much light) and large in dark conditions (allowing maximum possible light in). Around the iris is the white conjunctiva. As the upper lid normally rests just above the pupil, most of the conjunctiva is hidden. Regular blinking keeps the thin film of tears intact over the whole of the conjunctiva and cornea.

The relationship of these structures is shown in Figure 3.3. This diagram shows an imaginary cross section through the eye. Between the cornea and the lens is the anterior chamber. This is filled with fluid – the aqueous humour. The lens is controlled by the elastic suspensory ligaments and the circular ciliary muscle. When the ciliary muscle is relaxed, the suspensory ligaments pull the lens into a thin shape and the eye is focussed in the distance. When the ciliary muscle contracts the lens becomes a thickened, globular structure allowing focussing on very near objects. So to look at near objects, the ciliary muscles have to work hard.

Handbook of Retinal Screening in Diabetes, Roy Taylor
© 2006 John Wiley & Sons, Ltd

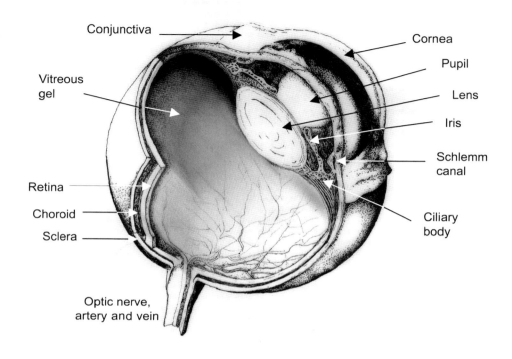

Conjunctiva

Cornea

Pupil

Vitreous
gel

Lens

Iris

Schlemm
canal

Retina

Choroid

Ciliary
body

Sclera

Optic nerve,
artery and vein

Figure 3.1   Cut-away three dimensional diagram of the eye. The flat picture of the retina seen in screening is in fact a representation of the inside of a sphere

Behind the lens is the main cavity of the eye, and this is filled with a dense jelly-like substance, the vitreous humour. Blood vessels run over the surface of the retina. Immediately behind the retina is a black layer – the choroid, a dark vascular structure. This black lining prevents reflection of light inside the eyeball. Behind the choroid is the sclera, a tough white layer which forms the outer covering of the eyeball.

The muscles which allow eye movements are attached to the sclera. The eyeballs sit in the orbits of the skull, cushioned by fatty tissue. The eye is a beautifully protected precision instrument.

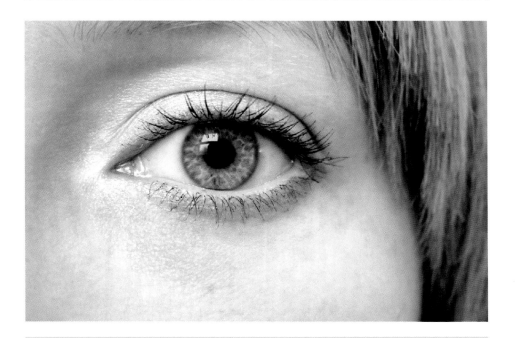

Figure 3.2 The eyeball is protected both by its position in the bony orbit of the skull and also by the eyelids. The upper eyelid normally is at rest just above the pupil, and the lower eyelid rests at the lower margin of the coloured iris. The tear film lubricates the movement of the eyelids over the cornea and conjunctiva and protects the delicate cells of these structures by keeping them moist

The retina

The retina is a transparent tissue of several different layers of cells. It is arranged in an upside-down fashion in that the light detecting cells (the photoreceptors) are deepest. Nerve fibres run vertically upwards and make contact with the nerve fibres which run across the surface of the retina to the optic nerve. Figure 3.4 shows retinal structure in a diagrammatical fashion.

Although the retina has a large surface area, all detailed vision is provided by one tiny area, the fovea. The fovea is in the centre of the macular region. It is important to understand this because of the potential effect of diabetes upon the fovea.

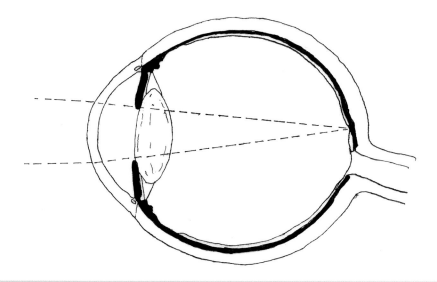

Figure 3.3 Horizontal cross section through the eye. This diagram shows the relationship of the structures to the incoming rays of light. The rays of light are refracted at the corneal surface and again in the lens so that they focus on the retina in the normal eye

The photoreceptor cells are of two main types. Rods detect any light, but cannot distinguish between colours. They account for the vast majority of photoreceptors. Cones detect colours and are found almost exclusively in the fovea.

Diabetic retinopathy

Diabetes causes problems in capillaries throughout the body but the problems can only be visualized in the retina. These tiny blood vessels have the job of channelling blood from arteries to veins. Because of this they allow the blood to deliver oxygen and food to tissues. There is a fine network of capillaries in all tissues. They are too small to be seen by the naked eye but give the retina its red colour because of the blood they contain.

The word 'retinopathy' just means disease of the retina. Diabetic retinopathy is a broad term which encompasses all the disorders of the retina caused

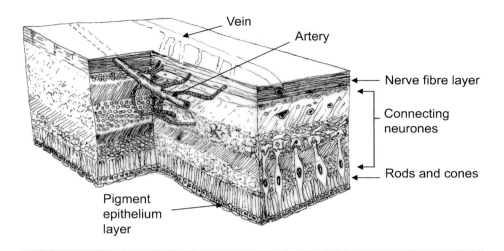

Vein

Artery

Nerve fibre layer

Connecting neurones

Rods and cones

Pigment epithelium layer

Figure 3.4 Microstructure of the retina. The light passes through the pupil and vitreous gel to impinge upon the surface of the retina. As the tissues of the retina are transparent, light passes through to reach the rods and cones which sit on the pigment epithelium in the inner, or deepest, part of the retina. There are two major capillary networks, one in the nerve fibre layer and one in the connecting neurone layers. Hypertension tends to cause haemorrhages in the former (which are therefore flame shaped when seen from above). Diabetes tends to cause haemorrhages in the latter (which appear round when seen from above as this layer of nerve fibres are running vertically)

by long-term high blood glucose levels. The particular problems which are caused by diabetes are illustrated in Figure 3.5. In order to discuss these several terms have to be defined.

Microaneurysms. These appear as small red dots on the retina. They are a result of ballooning of capillaries and are regarded as the earliest visible sign of diabetic retinopathy.

Blot haemorrhages. Rupture of small blood vessels in the deeper layers of the retina cause larger red lesions. They are approximately round but often with some irregularity of outline. The shape is determined by their position in the retina as they arise in the deeper layers where nerve fibres run perpendicular to the retinal surface. Although they look alarming to patients they do not cause functional disturbance.

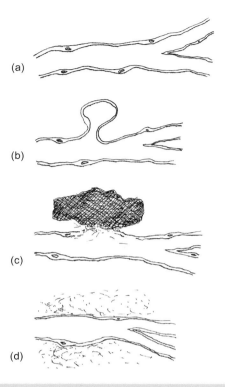

Figure 3.5 Diagrammatic representation of the different types of damage to capillaries in diabetic retinopathy. (a) A normal capillary. (b) A microaneurysm has formed by ballooning out of a weak part of the capillary wall. This appears as a dot to the observer. (c) A blot haemorrhage results from leakage of blood from a damaged capillary. This appears as a rounded blot to the observer. (d) An exudate results from the capillary wall being too leaky, and more plasma than usual escapes from the capillary. This appears as a white area, as the pressure causes blood to be squeezed from all surrounding capillaries

Exudates.   Leakage of plasma from capillaries causes yellow–white lesions with well-defined margins. Away from the macula region isolated exudates are not of particular concern. However, if they are within one disk diameter of the fovea the classification of the appearance changes from background to exudative maculopathy (see below).

Cotton wool spots.   Fuzzy pale areas on the retina occur due to swelling of the nerve fibres. This is caused by failure of the local capillary circulation and hence lack of oxygen and food delivery to the nerve fibres.

IRMA. 'Intra-retinal microvascular anomalies' takes so long to say that the abbreviation IRMA is always used. These are dilated small blood vessels and act as a sign of serious problems developing.

New vessels. When capillaries have become blocked the surrounding area is starved of oxygen and food. These tissues signal their plight using chemical messengers which stimulate the growth of new blood vessels. The new vessels grow towards the starving tissue in an attempt to supply it with oxygen and food. Unfortunately the new vessels are fragile and tend to grow into the space between the retina and the vitreous. When they rupture a large pre-retinal haemorrhage forms. This can be large enough to block all light detection and cause sudden loss of vision in that eye.

Background retinopathy. This is the presence of microaneurysms, blot haemorrhages or exudates. By itself it does not threaten sight. It indicates that there is an effect of diabetes upon the capillaries of the retina and shows that the person is at risk of developing other complications.

Proliferative retinopathy. This is said to be present when new vessels can be seen. The term refers to proliferation of the vascular endothelium into new blood vessels. When such changes are imminent, there may be irregularity of the diameter of veins, IRMA and/or cotton wool spots. Such changes are referred to as 'pre-proliferative' retinopathy.

Maculopathy. The macular region is at the posterior pole of the eye, close to the fovea. Maculopathy refers to visible changes of retinopathy close to the fovea. These changes can be picked up by screening and indicate the need for referral to an ophthalmologist. The concern is that there may be swelling (oedema) of the retina associated with the retinopathy. The macular oedema itself is not visible but can cause damage to the fovea which may be irreversible (see Chapter 9).

Other diabetes-associated changes in the eye

Cataracts

A cataract is cloudiness of the lens. There are many different appearances. There may be diffuse haziness, radial lines at the edge of the lens ('cartwheel') or central clumps of opacities.

Cataracts are common in older people. They occur 10–15 years earlier in people with diabetes. They can prevent adequate retinal images being obtained, and this is especially so with the central types.

Rubeosis iridis

New vessels can grow in the iris too. Here they can be seen by careful inspection. Immediate referral to an ophthalmologist is indicated. The reason for this is that the new vessels can grow to block the drainage of aqueous humour and cause an acute rise in pressure in the eye (acute glaucoma – see Chapter 12).

Mononeuropathies

Any nerve may be temporarily affected by diabetes, including the three nerves which control eye movements. The eyeball is moved by coordinated action of muscles in the orbit. If one nerve stops working, the eyeball on that side does not move as expected and double vision is caused. This is alarming for the patient but it is does not indicate permanent damage. A diabetologist needs to confirm the diagnosis by clinical examination and arrange an eye patch to cover the affected eye. This abolishes the troublesome double vision. The condition spontaneously improves in almost all cases over 2 months. It occurs in about one in every 1000 people with diabetes each year.

Further reading

1. Khaw, P.T. and Elkington, A.R. (1999) *ABC of Eyes*, 3rd edn, BMJ books.

Fact file

- The retina detects light.

- The iris regulates the amount of light entering the eye.

- The fovea is tiny but handles all detailed vision and all colour vision.

- The fovea is at the centre of the macular region.

- Diabetes can cause damage to retinal capillaries.

- Microaneurysms, blot haemorrhages and exudates occur in diabetic background retinopathy.

- Maculopathy refers to diabetes damage near the fovea (the macular region).

- Capillary leakage in the macular region may cause macular oedema.

- Venous irregularities and IRMA indicate pre-proliferative retinopathy.

- New vessels grow in response to failure of the microcirculation.

- New vessels are fragile and may rupture.

- Pre-retinal haemorrhage results from new vessels rupture.

- Cataracts are more common in people with diabetes.

4

The Need to Screen

Is blindness preventable?

From the patient's perspective, loss of sight is the most worrying potential consequence of diabetes. Any patient reading about their disease cannot help but be alarmed by the frequent references to blindness. Additionally, many older people will have heard tell of friends of friends who lost their sight due to diabetes. Indeed, it is the commonest cause of avoidable blindness in people between the ages of 16 and 64 years. Hard information upon this is sparse, but a thorough survey carried out in England and Wales showed that for the 12 month period between 1990 and 1991, 244 people lost their sight because of diabetes. It can be seen from Figure 4.1 that diabetes was the leading cause.

Retinopathy gradually develops in type 1 diabetes as time passes. It is unusual in the first 5 years, but thereafter more and more people show changes. After 25 years of type 1 diabetes, around 98 per cent of people have at least background retinopathy. By this time, almost 50 per cent of people will have had proliferative retinopathy and 15 per cent will have had macular oedema (Figure 4.2). It should be understood that these figures were gathered in the 1980s, and it is likely that the figures today are somewhat lower as explained below.

At the time of diagnosis of type 2 diabetes, around one third of people already have diabetic retinopathy to some degree. Even more strikingly, approximately 4 per cent of people have advanced retinopathy at the time of diagnosis. This emphasizes the crucial importance of all patients with type 2

Handbook of Retinal Screening in Diabetes, Roy Taylor
© 2006 John Wiley & Sons, Ltd

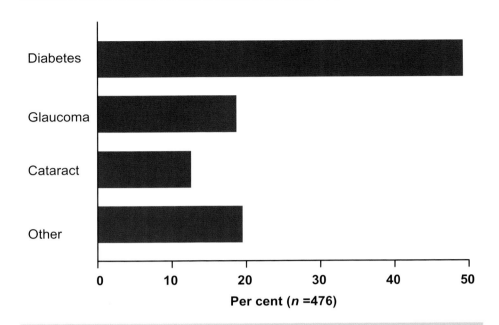

Figure 4.1 Causes of blindness in the working age population (16–64). The commonest causes of blindness were counted by analysing blindness registration certificates in England and Wales for the period 1990–1991 (data redrawn from Evans, J. *et al.* (1996) Blindness and partial sight in England and Wales 1990–1991. *Health Trends*, **28**:5–12)

diabetes having access to thorough retinal screening at the time of diagnosis. The prevalence of background retinopathy increases steadily with duration of disease, and around 20 per cent of all people with type 2 diabetes have proliferative retinopathy after 25 years of disease (Figure 4.3). Just as importantly, the prevalence of macular oedema steadily increases so that the same proportion (20 per cent) of people with type 2 diabetes are affected after 25 years of disease.

The length of time diabetes is present before blindness may occur is strikingly different between type 1 and type 2 diabetes. Figure 4.4 shows the distribution of duration of diabetes between 1998 and 2000 in Newcastle upon Tyne, UK. Each bar represents one person. Whereas 14 people had become blind within 10 years of diagnosis of type 2 diabetes, no-one with type 1 diabetes had become blind until almost 20 years after diagnosis. In this study it was found that blindness developed around 6 years after referral to the

Type 1 Diabetes

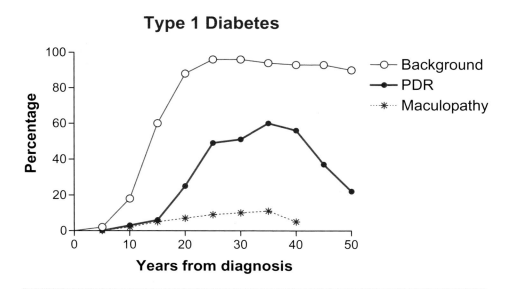

Figure 4.2 Change in the percentage of people having eye problems at different durations of type 1 diabetes (i.e. prevalence). The prevalence of background retinopathy, maculopathy and proliferative retinopathy are shown separately. The original data are from the Wisconsin Eye Study

ophthalmologist. However, the pattern of blindness is changing as a result of retinal screening. In 1985 there were six people under the age of 25 years who were blind, whereas at the time of the study in 2001 there were no blind people under the age of 35 years. The overall rate of blindness in diabetes was found to have fallen markedly. Screening is effective.

Can the progression of retinopathy be slowed?

It is now certain that good control of blood glucose can slow the rate of development of retinopathy. It can also slow the rate of progression of established retinopathy. Before 1994, this was a controversial matter, but clear information on type 1 diabetes was obtained from the Diabetes Control and Complications Trial (DCCT). The main results are shown in Figure 4.5. The difference between the group of people who had best possible blood glucose control and those who had ordinary care turned out to be striking. For the people who had no retinopathy at the start of the study, it can be seen that about 12 per cent showed retinal changes with ordinary control after 4 years, but in the group with good control it took 8 years for the same proportion to be affected (Figure 4.5).

Similar information about type 2 diabetes was obtained from the United Kingdom Prospective Diabetes Study (UKPDS). Figure 4.6 shows the effect of best possible control on the development of retinopathy. As in the DCCT, good control made a difference to the rate at which retinopathy worsened as the years went by. However, the UKPDS was able to show that control of blood pressure had a greater effect on the rate of progression of retinopathy than did tight control of blood glucose. This information has been very influential in bringing about a much more active approach to controlling blood pressure with advice to avoid salt in food and with prescription of one or more blood pressure-lowering drugs.

Taken together, these studies explain why the identification of background retinopathy is important. It changes the degree of urgency to achieve tight

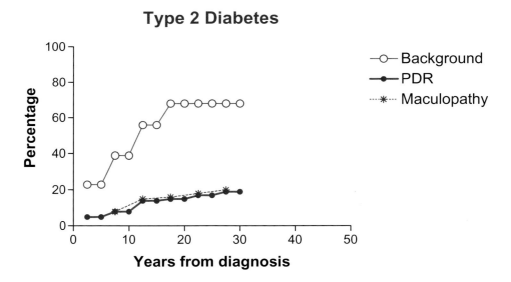

Figure 4.3 Change in the percentage of people having eye problems at different durations of type 2 diabetes. The prevalence of background retinopathy, maculopathy and proliferative retinopathy are shown separately. The original data are from the Wisconsin Eye Study

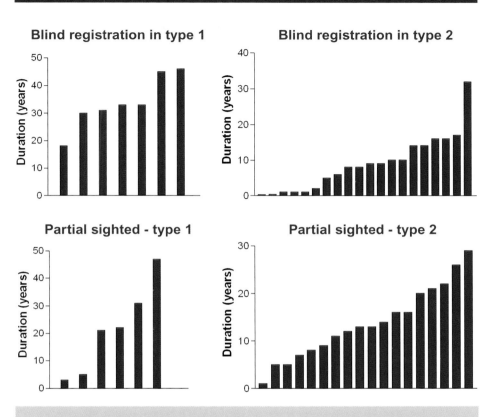

Figure 4.4 Duration of diabetes for each individual registered blind or partially sighted in Newcastle upon type 1998–2000

blood glucose levels and good blood pressure control. At a later stage, if exudative maculopathy is identified, the important treatment is to ensure that the doctor looking after the patient knows so that tight blood pressure control can urgently be arranged. It is for these reasons that retinal screening is an integral part of diabetes care. It should not operate as a free-standing service.

Detecting asymptomatic retinopathy

A major problem is that diabetic eye disease does not interfere with sight until it is advanced. Laser treatment can save sight, but only if it is used at an early

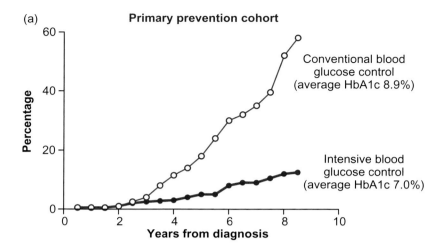

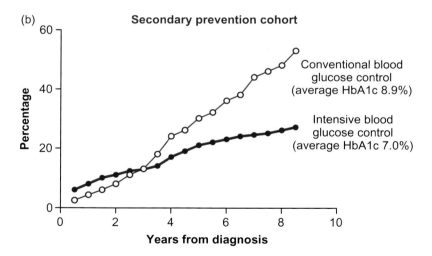

Figure 4.5   Percentages of people with type 1 diabetes showing significant worsening of retinopathy during the Diabetes Control and Complications Trial. (a) This shows the rate of change for people who had no retinopathy at the start of the study (called the primary prevention cohort) and (b) shows the rate of change for people who already had at least one complication of diabetes at the start of the study (secondary prevention cohort). Data replotted from Reference 6

stage. Because of this regular screening is necessary to detect when laser treatment may be required. Although people are still losing their sight because of diabetes, there is now clear evidence that repeated screening of populations leads to a fall in need for laser therapy. Data from Sweden has shown that the institution of a comprehensive screening program in Stockholm County resulted in a steady decrease in the annual incidence of blindness from just over 3 per 100 000 per year of the general population to around 0.2 per 100 000 per year over a 15 year period. The Newcastle data has also demonstrated that a comprehensive screening programme brings about a major fall in cases of blindness due to diabetes. Hence, it is now established that the majority of cases of blindness in diabetes are preventable.

This leads to three central questions about screening for diabetic retinopathy:

- Who? Everyone with diabetes.

- Where? Wherever most suitable for local conditions.

- How? Retinal imaging organized most suitably for local conditions.

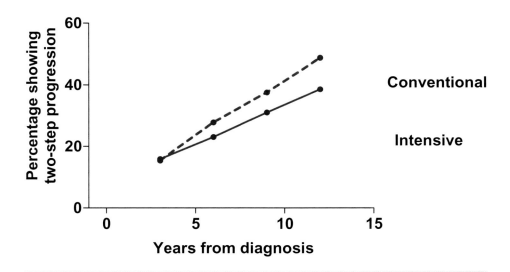

Figure 4.6 Rate of progression of retinopathy in groups of patients treated to achieve 'conventional' or 'intensive' blood pressure control. The data have been re-plotted from the UK Prospective Diabetes Study (Reference 4)

Digital retinal imaging is now widely accepted as the screening method of choice. In the UK the National Retinal Screening Project Group recommend that it is used. The challenge remains to establish screening systems which are effective, robust, and cost efficient in the circumstances of each health district. Given the wide variation between health districts in geography and facilities, it is likely that different approaches to the organization of screening will be required in different districts. Retinal screeners associated with the clinical diabetes service or optician-based systems are both in operation. Ophthalmoscopy by doctors or ophthalmologists can now be firmly excluded as a viable option for population screening.

The five principles of retinal screening

There are five issues of paramount importance:

1. to ensure regular screening is done;

2. to establish screening systems which are robust;

3. to make eye screening an integral part of diabetes care;

4. to involve the ophthalmologist in the planning and operation of local screening systems;

5. to establish ongoing quality control of the screening process.

The first and most important issue may seem odd on first reading. However, systematic screening by any means brings about a fall in blindness rates, even when relatively poor methods such as ophthalmoscopy have been used. The system set up in any one district must ensure that all people who may benefit are screened. Population coverage is the single most important factor which will determine future rates of diabetes blindness.

The second point is critical in that the service must not fall apart as soon as enthusiasm wanes or the person who set up the system moves away.

The third issue is often forgotten by those who do not have diabetes. The eye is one part of the whole body. Changes in the eye will inform treatment goals for blood pressure, lipids and blood glucose and knowledge of these will allow interpretation of observed retinal changes. Assessment of changes in the eye, kidney, nerve and foot allow the setting of annual goals for therapy. Retinal screening cannot be a free-standing activity, but must link closely with other aspects of diabetes care.

Fourthly, the main justification for screening is that the condition being sought is treatable. The criteria for referral to the ophthalmologist who specializes in diabetic eye disease need to be discussed locally. Arrangements must be made for fast-track assessment according to clinical urgency. By agreeing which appearances require routine assessment in the ophthalmology clinic and which require urgent assessment, timely treatment can be given and sight saved.

Finally, any screening system needs to be monitored continuously. Change of personnel, increased pressure upon the service and passage of time can all affect performance of human tasks, and collection of data on performance is most important in maintaining standards. A quality assurance system selects a percentage of images to be reassessed by a second, experienced screener. This is discussed below.

Quality assurance

The idea of quality assurance (QA) is well established in industry. A small sample of items coming off a production line will be carefully inspected. If the manufacturing process is not consistent then the faults will be identified. A sample which is too small may miss common faults, but a sample which is too large will be expensive and will slow production.

Quality assurance in retinal screening has been carried out as routine in some centres for many years. The experience in Newcastle upon Tyne, UK has been published. In this system the retinal screener tells the patient immediately the result of the screening and sends the result to the doctor caring for the person's diabetes. Twelve per cent of the images initially said to be abnormal are randomly selected for re-examination. Additionally, 2 per cent of the images said to be normal are similarly selected. This approach is necessary because otherwise the system would be flooded with normal images (around 70 per cent of any population of people with diabetes will have no retinopathy at any one time). The sample of images is examined by the consultant ophthalmologist. Then the initial and the second reports are compared. Over a 2 year period the sensitivity and specificity of detecting referable retinopathy were 88.3 per cent and 97.8 per cent respectively. Is this good enough? The current recommendations of the National Screening Committee state that sensitivity should each be over 80 per cent and specifity over 95 per cent – see Box 4.1 for explanation of these terms.

Box 4.1   Quality assurance

It has to be assumed that the second, more expert, assessment is correct. There can be four outcomes of screening:

- true negative – the image is normal and was reported by the screener as normal;

- true positive – the image shows retinopathy and was correctly reported by the screener;

- false negative – the image shows retinopathy but was reported by the screener as normal;

- false positive – the image is normal but was reported by the screener as showing retinopathy.

There are two separate questions to be answered. The more important is whether the screener reports all the images which require referral correctly. The second is whether the screener picks up the earliest signs of retinopathy in all cases.

The possibilities can be more simply understood as a table. This shows the possible outcomes of examining any one image in respect of detecting all referable retinopathy:

	Screener says refer	Screener says referral not needed
Expert says refer	True positive	False negative
Expert says referral not needed	False positive	True negative

Sensitivity

Sensitivity refers to the detection of all images requiring referral in the example above. For a series of images assessed over a period of time it is defined as:

$$\frac{\text{True positives}}{\text{True positives} + \text{False negatives}} \times 100$$

Try working out what the sensitivity would be if a screener correctly referred 45 patients in a year but missed five cases the expert said should be referred.

Specificity

Specificity refers to the accuracy of detection of images requiring referral in the example above. It would not be effective if a screener consistently over-referred patients as the ophthalmologist would be unable to deal rapidly with cases truly requiring referral. For a series of images assessed over a period of time it is defined as:

$$\frac{\text{True negatives}}{\text{True negatives} + \text{False positives}} \times 100$$

Try working out what the specificity would be if a screener correctly reported 4000 images which did not require referral in a year, but reported a further 1000 images as requiring referral which the expert said did not require referral.

The percentage of patients selected for review of images depends upon the exact question being tested by the QA and also on its affordability. In the UK, it has been suggested that all images showing any change associated with diabetes should be QA'ed along with a proportion of normal images. Whether this heavy-handed approach will be affordable by Primary Care Trusts remains to be seen. It is doubtful that such an intense system of checking of results is necessary for best practice, and some modification of the Newcastle upon Tyne approach may be the likeliest long-term practice.

You should not be alarmed at the idea of not correctly classifying every image. If two experts were to report on a series of images it is likely that they will disagree on a proportion of them. Indeed, the experts may disagree with themselves if asked to report on the same image on two different days. There will always be a small number of borderline cases which could reasonably be classified either way. The referral guidelines take account of this to ensure patient safety. However, the vital point is that it should be rare for a definitely referable appearance to be misclassified.

History of the development of retinal screening by photography-based systems in the UK

The first demonstration of successful retinal photography was carried out in Cardiff. However, the prevailing expert opinion was that it would never be satisfactory for screening. At that time, screening was carried out using the ophthalmoscope in diabetes clinics, often irregularly.

To test whether screening using the 'non-mydriatic' camera was as good as ophthalmology, a study was carried out in Newcastle upon Tyne between 1986 and 1988. The camera was mounted in a mobile unit in order to be able to use the expensive equipment every day, by driving it to whichever diabetes clinics was running. This study demonstrated that Polaroid retinal photography was much better than ophthalmoscopy with mydriasis in detecting maculopathy and was at least as good in detecting new vessels. A major observation was that small pupils prevented adequate photography in 1 in 20 people and as a result routine mydriasis with tropicamide has been recommended ever since. As a direct result of this study, together with the use of Newcastle upon Tyne data, the British Diabetic Association was able to attract substantial charitable funding (from the Allied Dunbar Foundation) which was used to set up 10 other mobile retinal screening units in other parts of the country.

These mobile units did well. Over 64 000 eye screening episodes were recorded to September 1994, 76.5 per cent of them in a primary care setting and 23.5 per cent as part of hospital based screening; 5.6 per cent of those screened were referred to the ophthalmologist and 1.2 per cent of those screened or 22 per cent of those referred received laser therapy.

The major development in the last decade has been the move to establish comprehensive screening programmes – in other words to ensure that everyone with diabetes in a District receives annual screening. This is the only way to make a major impact upon the rate of diabetes blindness in the population.

Fact file

- Diabetes is the leading cause of blindness in the working age population of the UK.

- In type 1 diabetes, 98 per cent have at least background retinopathy after 25 years.

- In type 1 diabetes, around 50 per cent of people have developed proliferative retinopathy after 25 years.

- In type 1 diabetes, around 15 per cent of people with type 1 diabetes have developed exudative maculopathy after 25 years.

- At the time of diagnosis, one third of people with type 2 diabetes have diabetic retinopathy.

- In type 2 diabetes, around 20 per cent of people have developed proliferative retinopathy after 25 years.

- In type 2 diabetes, around 20 per cent of people will have developed exudative maculopathy after 25 years.

- Retinopathy causes no visual disturbance until it is advanced.

- Laser therapy is most effective when used early for sight threatening retinopathy.

- All people with diabetes need to have retinal screening annually.

- The organization of the District screening system is important.

- QA needs to be built into the screening system.

Further reading

1. http://www.dtu.ox.ac.uk/index.html?maindoc=/ukpds/
2. http://medweb.bham.ac.uk/easdec/prevention/UKPDS%20study.htm
3. **http://www.nsd.scot.nhs.uk/services/drs/**
4. 'Tight blood pressure control and risk of macrovascular and microvascular complications in type 2 diabetes: UKPDS 38'. BMJ 1998;317:703–13.
5. http://diabetes.niddk.nih.gov/dm/pubs/control/
6. DCCT (1993) The effect of intensive treatment of diabetes on the development and progression of long-term complications in insulin-dependent diabetes mellitus. The Diabetes Control and Complications Trial Research Group. *New England Journal of Medicine*, **329**:977–986.
7. Pandit, R.J. and Taylor, R. (2002) 'Quality assurance in screening for sight-threatening diabetic retinopathy'. *Diabetic Medicine*, **19**:285–291.
8. Arun, C.S., Ngugi, N. and Taylor, R. (2003) 'Effectiveness of screening in preventing blindness due to diabetic retinopathy'. *Diabetic Medicine*, **20**:186–90.
9. Arun, C.S. *et al.* (2006) Establishing an ongoing quality assurance in retinal screening programme. *Diabetic Medicine*, in press.

5

Practical Screening

Important first steps

The retinal screening examination is a clinical procedure governed by important considerations.

Confidentiality is paramount. No personal information of any kind can be allowed to be divulged to others. A person's medical condition is private information and no aspect of it may be discussed in a public place or with any person outside the health care team. Retinal screeners are privileged to know who has diabetes in a community and this information is strictly confidential. Nothing learned during the screening episode may be repeated outside the health care team.

Are you sure you are screening the right person? Identity must be confirmed before screening. A person may be invited from the waiting area by calling the name. Then, in private, the full name needs to be confirmed together with date of birth or address.

Does the person understand what is to be done? Even though a leaflet describing the screening procedure may have been sent to them with the appointment, you cannot assume that the information has been understood. An example of the form of words which may be used is given on page 58.

Handbook of Retinal Screening in Diabetes, Roy Taylor
© 2006 John Wiley & Sons, Ltd

Measuring visual acuity

How well the eye can see details is tested using the Snellen chart. The person must be comfortably seated 6 m away from the chart which must be adequately illuminated. Each eye is tested separately to obtain the 'best corrected visual acuity'. This means that errors of refraction (short or long sightedness) are corrected. The purpose of the test is to see how well the retina is functioning. In order to do this the person should wear their distance glasses if worn. A pinhole device is used if visual acuity is 6/9 or less as this corrects refractive errors.

The effect of refractive errors (short- or long-sightedness) is illustrated in Figure 5.1 and the reason why a simple pinhole can correct these is explained in Figure 5.2.

Procedure

1. Explain what is to be done.

2. Always test the right eye first and record the result to avoid mixing up the results from each eye.

3. Ask the person to read out the letters starting from the top.

4. The last line to be correctly read is recorded.

5. If the visual acuity is 6/9 or worse then use the pinhole and test again.

6. Record if the reading was done with glasses or pinhole.

7. If the person is unable to read the top letter of the chart, seat them 3 m from the chart. Retest and record as 3/60 etc.

8. If no letters can be read at 3 m, record whether or not light can be seen by the eye.

Interpretation of visual acuity measurement

Various factors can affect the result such as anxiety, any feeling of hurry and other psychological factors. It is conventionally accepted that a true deterio-

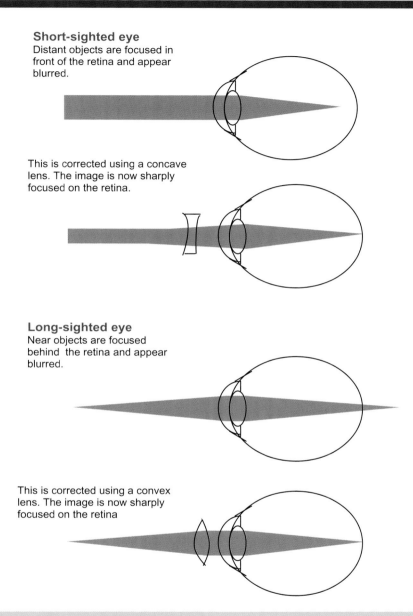

Short-sighted eye
Distant objects are focused in
front of the retina and appear
blurred.

This is corrected using a concave
lens. The image is now sharply
focused on the retina.

Long-sighted eye
Near objects are focused
behind the retina and appear
blurred.

This is corrected using a convex
lens. The image is now sharply
focused on the retina

Figure 5.1 Refractive errors – the diagrams show what happens to a ray of light entering the eye. Light is focused in front of the retina in a short-sighted eye. Use of a concave lens causes the light to diverge slightly, and the image is now in focus on the retina. The image is focused behind the retina in a long-sighted eye, and a convex lens corrects this

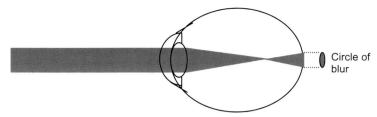

In a short-sighted eye, the focal point is in front of the fovea and a circle of blur is created at the fovea.

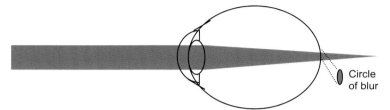

In a long-sighted eye, the focal point is behind the fovea and again a circle of blur is created at the fovea.

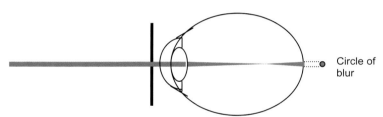

In a short-sighted eye, the pinhole makes the circle of blur much smaller at the fovea, and the image is sharper (but dimmer as less light gets into the eye – keep that chart brightly lit!).

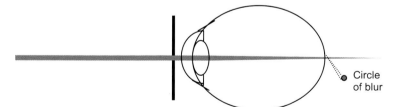

Also in a long-sighted eye, the pinhole makes the circle of blur much smaller at the fovea, and the image is sharper.

Figure 5.2 How the pinhole works – For both short- and long-sighted eyes, the image is out of focus on the retina as a larger, blurred image. This is called the circle of blur. By restricting the diameter of the ray of light entering the eye the circle of blur is decreased in size and the image appears sharper. As less light is entering the eye it is important that the object (Snellen chart) is brightly lit

ration in vision has occurred if there is a difference of more than two lines from the previous screening test (e.g. 6/06 to 6/12). A difference of one line (e.g. 6/06 to 6/09) has be to described as no clear difference from last time.

If a deterioration in visual acuity cannot be explained by any known condition such as forgotten glasses or cataract, then referral is required to exclude the possibility of macular oedema (see Chapter 9). Even though this possibility is remote in clinical practice, caution demands an appropriate examination.

Instilling eye drops

Mydriasis refers to the act of dilating the pupil. The mydriatic eye drop used in screening programmes is tropicamide (0.5 per cent or 1 per cent strength). Retinal screeners must understand tropicamide's effects, the legal basis for its use and how to administer the eye drops. The pupil requires to be dilated to obtain the best possible image of the retina in most adults. Over the age of 50 years it becomes progressively less likely that a good image could be obtained without mydriasis. However, in adolescents it is likely that good images may be obtained without the use of mydriasis. The retinal screener will normally be given the discretion to decide on whether eye drops may not be required in the under 25 year age group.

Mydriatic drops should not be instilled until after visual acuity has been measured.

Tropicamide

In the UK eye drops may be administered by any staff trained to do so. Normally the doctor in charge of the screening programme would have signed a document to say that eye drops may be administered as appropriate for retinal screening. The local arrangements for storage of tropicamide or any other drops must be adequate to allow security and monitoring of stocks.

Tropicamide is a drug and its actions and side effects must be understood by all screeners.

Action

Tropicamide causes dilatation of the pupil by temporary paralysis of the circular muscle around the iris (sphincter pupillae muscle). It diffuses rapidly through the cornea to reach the iris. Adequate papillary dilatation is usually achieved in 10 minutes and the effect starts to wane after about 2 hours.

Side effects

Administration of the eye drop causes a stinging feeling (similar to that of getting some soap in the eye). Patients must be warned in advance of this effect.

The main side effect is blurring of vision. This occurs because the muscle of the ciliary body is also affected to a modest extent. Focusing on near objects is most affected, and the effect can be expected to last about 2 hours. Some people are more affected than others.

Sensitivity to bright light occurs because the pupil is held open. This is particularly troublesome on sunny days, especially in snowy conditions. Patients should be advised to bring along sunglasses to wear after screening to avoid being dazzled. Because of all the potential effects on vision patients should not drive for 2 hours after administration of tropicamide.

Contraindications to tropicamide use

The single contraindication to tropicamide use is the need to engage in detailed visual work or driving immediately after screening.

Safety

Tropicamide is a safe eye drop in general. In particular it is the case that tropicamide does not cause acute glaucoma (see Chapter 14). It can be used in people with glaucoma on medical treatment, in people after surgical treatment of glaucoma and those people with a family history of glaucoma. This is not necessarily the case if mydriatic drops stronger than tropicamide are used or when eye drops are used in combination.

The earliest kind of intra-ocular artificial lens implant was balanced against the back of the pupil and dilatation of the pupil could cause displacement. However, these implants have not been used since 1985.

A red eye, current use of other eye drops or creams, and recent eye surgery are not medical contraindications to tropicamide use. However, the patient may be uncomfortable at the thought of instilling tropicamide drops even though it would be perfectly safe. In such a case arrangements should be made to postpone the screening.

Instilling tropicamide

1. Explain the need for eye drops and obtain the person's verbal consent.

2. Check the drug name and concentration on minim and confirm that the expiry date has not passed.

3. Position the head looking up to the ceiling and ask the person to look up and to the left. The right eye is thus looking away from the site of administration (Figure 5.3).

4. Gently pull down the right lower lid.

5. Instil one drop of tropicamide into the trough formed by the inside of the lower lid and the conjunctiva.

6. Ask the person to blink. This speeds the spreading of the eye drop over the conjunctiva and cornea.

7. Provide a tissue to dab away excess tropicamide which may have spilt onto the face during blinking.

8. Repeat for the left eye, using a separate disposable minim of tropicamide to avoid any possibility of cross-infection.

9. Record the administration of tropicamide in accordance with local documentation.

10. Wait approximately 10 minutes for dilatation to occur.

Other eye drops

In most screening programmes individuals whose pupils do not dilate adequately with one drop of tropicamide (0.5 or 1 per cent) would be given a second dose of tropicamide (1 per cent). Other programmes use phenyle-

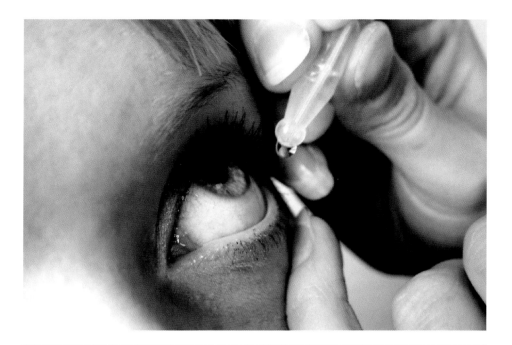

Figure 5.3 Instilling eye drops – it is important that the subject knows what is to happen in advance and that the drop will cause a 'soap in the eye' feeling. The patient is asked to look up and away from the site of administration with the aim of placing the drop in the conjunctival sac

phrine but, if authorized, this strong mydriatic must be used with great care and local guidelines followed.

In the past it was thought helpful to reverse the mydriasis after examination using pilocarpine eye drops, which constrict the pupil. This practice has no sound basis and may cause serious complications. Pilocarpine has no place in a retinal screening programme.

Obtaining the image

1. Check that the person knows what is to be done.

2. Sit the patient in front of the camera and position his/her chin on the chin rest (Figure 5.4).

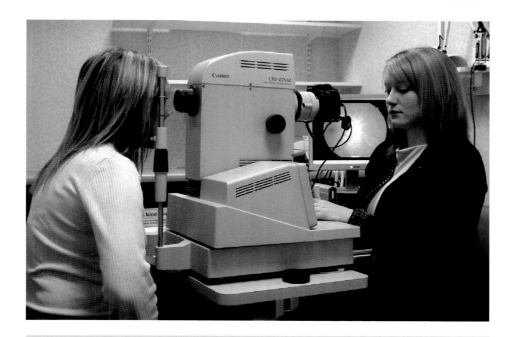

Figure 5.4 The subject should be sitting comfortably with their chin on the chin rest and their forehead against the head rest. The operator should also be sitting comfortably

3. Slide the camera unit to the eye to be imaged (always right eye first) by moving the joystick left or right.

4. Press the alignment switch to display the external eye image on the video monitor. The pupil of the eye to be imaged should be centred on the pupil alignment mark seen on the monitor.

5. Focus by slowly moving the joystick forwards or backwards.

6. Press the alignment switch to display the retinal image. If the corneal reflection dots are absent, further adjustment of the joystick is required. If the split lines are absent then the height or left–right adjustments of the joystick are incorrect.

7. Align the split lines by rotating the fine focusing knob. If at any subsequent point the split lines become separated then the focusing knob must be readjusted.

8. Ask your subject to look straight at the green flashing light within the camera, following it if necessary.

9. The fixation light should be moved until the retinal image seen on the monitor is correctly aligned with the optic disc central for the first image capture.

10. When the corneal reflection dots are sharp, the split lines are aligned and the correct area of retina is displayed the exposure button may be pressed.

11. Is the image technically satisfactory? If so, proceed to take an image with fovea central on the picture.

12. Repeat the procedure for the left eye.

Examining the image

Can you rely on your vision?

There is a difference between looking at a picture and systematically checking each part of it. This is why 'eye witness accounts' are notoriously unreliable. Groups of people shown a video clip of an incident and questioned about it afterwards will give very different reports: there were two men who broke the window / there were three men; one was blond / one was dark; they ran off to the left / right; there were no people close to them / there were some people close by, etc.

The explanation for this lies in how the brain interprets very limited information and fills in the gaps. At any one time only the very small area projected onto the fovea can see fine detail and colour. Our eyes move to scan only a small sample of a scene, and our brains literally make up the rest – from experience. There are no colour receptors outside the fovea, and the vast majority of our visual fields can only see black, white and grey. Yet we imagine we can see colour all round (see Further reading).

This is important to understand when considering how to examine a retinal image. Is it normal or are there some abnormalities? We must consciously direct our eyes to each part of the image. For this reason all descriptions of retinal images in this book follow a fixed order:

- optic disc

- then vessels

- then retina section by section.

Only in this way is it possible to be certain of obtaining all useful information in the short time available during busy screening sessions.

Look at any image in Chapter 6. What do you see? How can you tell whether it is normal? After reading Chapter 3 you will recognize the major structures – the optic disc, blood vessels and the retina itself. Each of these must be looked at in turn.

Disc

Look at Figure 6.1. The disc is a pale yellow in parts, and this merges into a pinkish colour. Such variation in colour is normal, although any pinkish area needs to be scrutinized carefully to ensure that it is not made up of a blush of fine new vessels. There is no sign of this. There are some small vessels on the disc, but these are single and are going in purposeful directions (quite different from new vessels as seen in Chapter 10).

Vessels

Both arteries and veins can be seen. The arteries are smaller in diameter and lighter in colour often with a bright reflection along their length. The veins are darker in colour and wider than the arteries at any comparable point. Starting with the main vein going up from the disc, follow it along its length. It gets gradually thinner as more branches leave the main vessel. It is generally smooth in outline, with fairly constant diameter over each segment. Note the pale line which can be seen within the vein especially at the last junction before the edge of the image. This is merely a light reflection artefact and is entirely normal. Now double back and look at each of the branches in turn. Each of the veins diminishes in size and none have loops or any tangled new vessels arising from them. Repeat the process in the lower half of the image.

Retina

The colour of the retina varies with some lighter patches merging with the background pink especially towards the disc. This is a phenomenom of light reflection from the retina, although normal variability in retinal thickness can also contribute. Close to the left-hand margin there are some areas which appear dark. Again, this is well within the normal variability of pigmentation. Now scrutinize each segment of the retina in turn. It is convenient to use the vessels as boundaries between segments. Above the disk, the artery defines an area – which is unremarkable. Next door, there is an area between artery and vein. In this area there is a normal streaky appearance due to nerve fibres running in parallel towards the disc. Continue to move clockwise round the image looking at each segment in turn.

Finally, look at the centre of the macula region. In this image the fovea does not stand out as a distinct dot, but is in the centre of the darker red area. It is this colour because of the greater concentration of capillaries.

If you have trouble reading any image a further question must be asked: is the image assessable? If the vessels are not clear beyond the third branching, or if less than two thirds of the retinal area is visible, then the image has to be considered inadequate.

Exhausted after one image? With practice an image can be thoroughly and systematically examined in around 20 seconds, and with experience the normal variants discussed above can be confidently set aside.

Explaining the results of screening

Good communication is the essence of good diabetes care. Diabetes is unusual amongst medical conditions in that doctors and nurses do not do the treatment – rather the individual has to do the treatment for themselves, day after day. Effective communication of all the necessary information is the business of all members of the diabetes team. The person with diabetes needs to have full information about their condition. In the case of eye screening it is important that the result of screening is communicated at the time of the screening session. Not only does this relieve anxiety but also it helps to ensure that the person returns for their next screening visit.

Experience has shown that trained retinal screeners can classify the vast majority of retinal images accurately and with confidence. After more than

6 months of experience a screener may be uncertain about one in every few hundred images. New and unknown appearances will continue to occur at a very low frequency through an entire career and advice must be sought appropriately. Hence, the screener will be in a position to inform the patient fully about their retinal appearances in most cases, and will have to give a provisional report on very few with a promise of further information to follow.

The operation of the quality assurance system does not interfere with the process of patient care. Patients must be informed about the quality assurance system, and this would normally be done in the information leaflet sent out with the appointment. Providing that the retinal screener has been adequately trained and providing that the systematic method of examining images is consistently used, the number of occasions that a revised interpretation of retinal appearances will be required will be very few indeed.

A standard form of words will normally be used to explain the appearances.

- 'There are no signs of diabetes affecting the eyes. A further test in one year will be important.'

- 'There are some signs of diabetes in the eyes, but these are stable. There is no immediate risk to the eyesight. However, it will be important to aim for good control of both blood glucose and blood pressure. You should discuss this with your doctor.'

- 'There are some signs of diabetes in the eyes and these appear stable. It will be important to be certain that there is no further change and a further appoint will be made for your eyes to be screened in 6 months time.'

- 'There are changes of diabetes in the eyes and these do need to be fully assessed by an eye specialist. An appointment will be arranged for you to be seen in the next few weeks/months.'

Most people will benefit from seeing their own retinal images to be able to understand exactly what is being talked about. A moment pointing out normal retina on the one hand or lesions on the other can be of enormous benefit to patients.

The suggested forms of words will not necessarily be satisfactory for all patients. Individuals differ in their response both to basic information and to words. With experience satisfactory communication of results with virtually all patients will be possible. This is a people-handling skill, but the initial consideration for a retinal screener is that they should be confident of their interpretation of the retinal appearances.

Organization of a district screening system

The essence of retinal screening can readily be described: a call and recall appointment system, examination by a trained retinal screener, feedback of the result to the patient and continuous assessment of the performance of the system.

The appointment system organizes a screening visit. The result of screening is immediately communicated to the patient. This is vital both for the patient's peace of mind and also to maximize the chance of the person returning for screening on the next occasion. The result is also communicated to the doctor caring for the patient's diabetes to inform decisions about blood glucose and blood pressure control. If necessary referral to the ophthalmologist is initiated. In some centres this is done directly by the retinal screener and in others it is done via the doctor responsible for the person's diabetes.

In the background, two additional systems operate. Firstly, the QA system samples sets of images, provides a second reading of the image and generates sensitivity and specificity data (see Chapter 4). Secondly, the attendances for screening are logged and information on completeness of population coverage is acquired.

The basic organization is independent of the local arrangements for delivery of the screening. This may be done in a fixed unit, perhaps as part of the diabetes centre, in a mobile screening unit or in an opticians shop. Local factors are highly important in determining what will work best in view of local facilities and geography.

Links with your ophthalmologist

It is most important that there is a close working relationship between the local consultant ophthalmologist who specializes in diabetic retinopathy and the diabetes eye screening service. The general indications for referral are nationally agreed, but local agreements on detail will always be important. The dialogue should extend to sending copy of any difficult image directly to the ophthalmologist for comment. Such cases might include previously lasered eyes in which the screener was uncertain whether the current appearances represent any further cause for concern, especially if the patient has been discharged back to routine screening. This communication can save unnecessary referrals.

By minimizing the number of unnecessary referrals and by allowing discharge of patients stable after laser therapy, it is possible to decrease waiting times for all referrals. The clear benefit of an effective diabetes eye screening programme for ophthalmology has been demonstrated over the last decade.

The classification of retinal appearances and definition of need for referral is shown in Table 5.1. This classification has been agreed in the UK by a group of diabetologists and ophthalmologists (see further reading, reference 3).

Further reading

1. Gregory, R.L. (1998) *Eye and Brain: The Psychology of Seeing*, Oxford University Press, Oxford.
2. Maguire, P. (2000) *Communication Skill for Doctors*, Arnold, London.
3. Harding, S. *et al.* (2003) Grading and disease management in national screening for diabetic retinopathy in England and Wales. *Diabetic Medicine*, **20**:965–971.

Table 5.1 Retinopathy grading system proposed for the National Retinopathy Screening Programme. All images can be graded by use of the RMP score (e.g. R1, M0, P0 for background retinopathy). In clinical practice it is very useful to subdivide R1 into early background (microaneurysms, blot haemorrhages one or two exudates away from macula) and moderate background (many haemorrhages or exudates). The latter are at high risk of progression

Retinopathy (R)

R0	None	
R1	Background	microaneurysm(s) retinal haemorrhage(s) ± any exudate
R2	Pre-proliferative	venous beading venous loop or reduplication intraretinal microvascular abnormality (IRMA) multiple deep, round or blot haemorrhages (if cotton wool spots – careful search for above)
R3	Proliferative	new vessels on disc new vessels elsewhere pre-retinal or vitreous haemorrhage pre-retinal fibrosis ± tractional retinal detachment

Maculopathy (M)

M0	None	one or two microaneuryms or blot haemorrhage permitted in 1 DD of fovea (see below)
M1	Referable	exudate within 1 disc diameter (DD) of the center of the fovea circinate or group of exudates within the macula microaneurysms or haemorrhages within 1 DD of the centre of the fovea only if associated with a best VA of ≤6/12 (if no stereo)

Photocoagulation (P)

P0	None	
P1	Previous laser	

Fact file

- Absolute patient confidentiality must be maintained.

- Confirm identity before screening.

- Confirm understanding of procedure before screening.

- VA measurement is susceptible to error unless very carefully done.

- Tropicamide eye drops dilate the pupil.

- Tropicamide acts within 10 minutes and lasts about 2 hours.

- Driving is not advised for 2 hours after tropicamide.

- Additional use of phenylephrine eye drops must follow local guidelines.

- Never use pilocarpine to 'reverse' mydriasis.

- Examine each retinal image systematically: disc, vessels, retina.

- Explain the results of screening in words appropriate for the individual.

- A quality assurance system checks on effectiveness and efficiency.

- Sensitivity in a QA system is a measure of picking up all abnormailities.

- Specificity in a QA system is a measure of avoiding reports of abnormalities when they are none.

- Sensitivity should be over 80 per cent and specificity over 95 per cent.

- Close working links with your ophthalmologist are important.

6
Normal Retinal Appearances

Normal retinas come in a wide range of colours and patterns, with variable patterns of arteries and veins. Some young people have eyes which sparkle, and they tend to have sparkling retinas too. This light reflection pattern sometimes makes examination difficult. Others have relatively thin retinas, allowing the choroid circulation to be visible and giving rise to concern about possible abnormal blood vessels. To make life even more interesting for the retinal screener a variety of artefacts may occur. A blink at the wrong split second results in a white out. Slight narrowing of the eyelids causes a bright blur at the edge of the image. Eye lashes in the way of the flash cause pale stripes, and bushy eyebrows can produce pop-art designs.

Fortunately, most artefacts can be easily recognized by their characteristics, even though the range of normal variants is very wide indeed. The images in this chapter display this range although some also show features of diabetic retinopathy.

Handbook of Retinal Screening in Diabetes, Roy Taylor
© 2006 John Wiley & Sons, Ltd

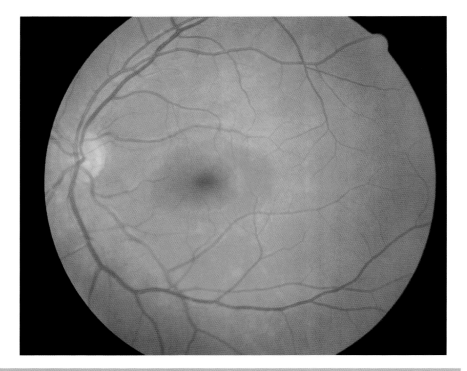

Figure 6.1   Light reflection artefact

Disc

The optic disc is of normal, pale colour. Only the temporal margin of the disc is clearly defined. The retina fades into the disc nasally, and this is a normal appearance. The small vessels on the disc are running in purposeful directions.

Vessels

The veins are moderately dilated (ratio more than 3:2 compared with the arteries). In the upper field the veins are obviously of even calibre, but at first inspection this does not appear to be the case for the inferior temporal vein. However, light reflection artefacts are present beside this vein, most obvious just below the disc. These account for the apparent moth-eaten appearance of the vein.

Retina

Examining each section of the retina, starting just above the disc and moving clockwise, it is clear that the retinal colour varies. It is pink just above the disc, paler above the macula region and darkish towards the temporal margin. This variation is well within normal. The very pale pattern which almost circles the fovea is a light reflection artefact. Note that it has an indistinct, flocculated pattern which is totally different from exudates or cotton wool spots. The pale circle just to the right of the fovea is a reflection of the camera bulb.

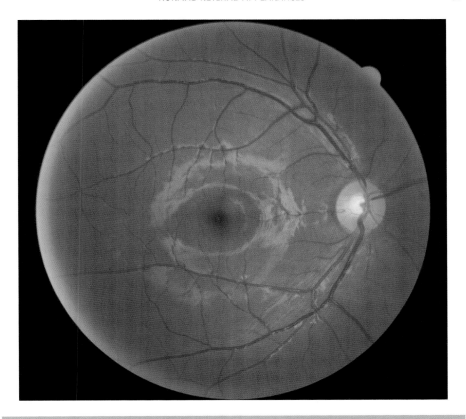

Figure 6.2 Light reflection artefact

Disc

The disc margins are clearly defined all round. The pale area in the centre of the disc is the optic cup which is normal size (i.e. less than half the disc diameter). The small vessels which can be seen on the disc are all single and not tortuous.

Vessels

The veins are normal in calibre (approximately 3 : 2 compared with the arteries. There are pale streaks and dots scattered along the veins together with pale patches on the retina near the veins. The appearances are typical of reflection artefacts, most often seen in the eyes of younger people. In clinical practice a confident diagnosis can be made by comparing with the disc centred image of the same eye in which the pattern of reflection will be different because of the different angle of light striking the retina.

Retina

Just above the disc there is an elongated, poorly defined pale area. Moving clockwise, the retina is unremarkable until the area just below the disc is reached. There are several small, poorly defined areas. Pale streaks can be seen running down from the disc at about 7 o'clock to the disc. Other pale areas are scattered over the peripheral retina. The background colour of the retina displays the normal variation in shade of pink. The most striking feature is the pale incomplete rings and flocculated pale patches around the macula region. These are all reflection artefacts (again, see Figures 7.2 and 8.4). There is a normal point reflection of light from the centre of the fovea.

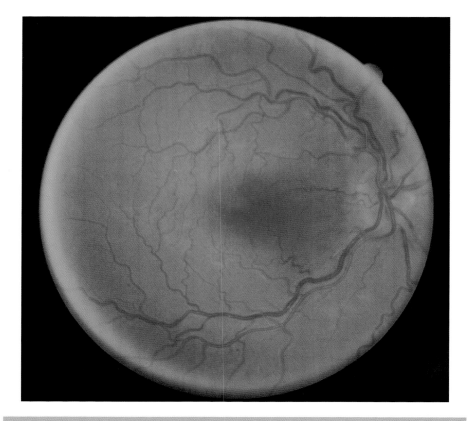

Figure 6.3   Tortuous vessels

Disc

The disc is poorly defined but is of normal pale colour. The optic cup cannot be seen. Normal small vessels – single, non-tortuous – are present.

Vessels

Both veins and arteries follow a wavy course. This is so throughout the course of most vessels. The appearance might be thought to suggest new vessel formation, but each vessel heads in a purposeful direction and is single. Light reflection artefacts on the vessels can be seen.

Retina

The colour of the retina appears to vary from yellow to pink in the light of the flash. This is normal. However, systematic examination of the retina shows that there are some microaneurysms present. There are two exudates, one near the temporal border of the image, close to some microaneurysms.

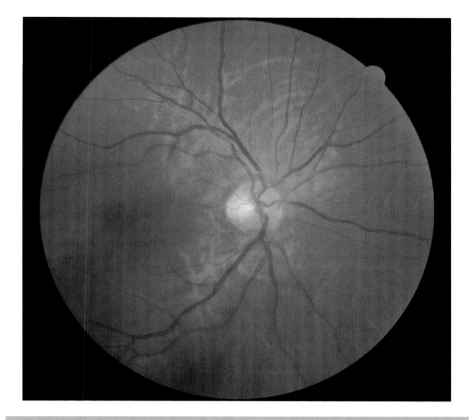

Figure 6.4 Tiger striping

Disc

The margins are unremarkable and a small optic cup can be seen. The small vessels on the disc are single and head in purposeful directions.

Vessels

The veins are moderately engorged (ratio close to 2:1). The pale streak overlying the vein just above the disc is a reflection artefact.

Retina

The background colour of the retina is striking, broad pale lines separating normal but darkish retina. This variation in distribution of pigmentation is unusual but does not signify any disease process. When this 'tiger striping' is present particular care is required to examine the retina for lesions of diabetic retinopathy. The retina is normal in this image.

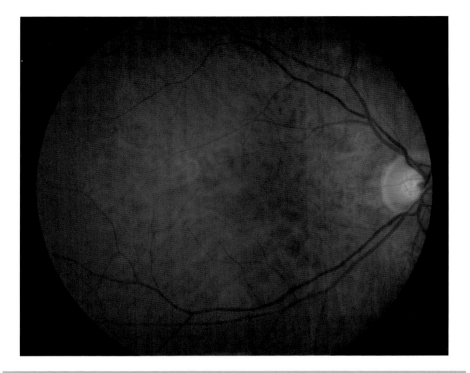

Figure 6.5   Tiger striping

Disc

The visible disc margin is normal. The optic cup can be distinguished in the centre of the disc as a pale area. The small vessels on the disc are each single and running in purposeful directions.

Vessels

The veins are of normal calibre. Following each out to the edge of the image shows no abnormality. One disc diameter above the disc it can be seen that the vein appears to 'disappear' behind the artery. This arterio venous nipping or crossing-change raises a question of high blood pressure, but careful examination of all other crossing points of vein and artery are normal.

Retina

The variation in background colour of the retina is striking. Examining the retina section by section in a clockwise manner gives an overall impression of multiple pale bands with darker, pigmented retina in between. This is referred to as a tiger-striped retina and is a normal variant. On such a film more time requires to be taken to inspect each area of the retina in turn to detect any lesions of diabetes. On this film there is a single microaneurysm at 10 o'clock to the fovea, approximately two thirds of the distance to the edge of the image.

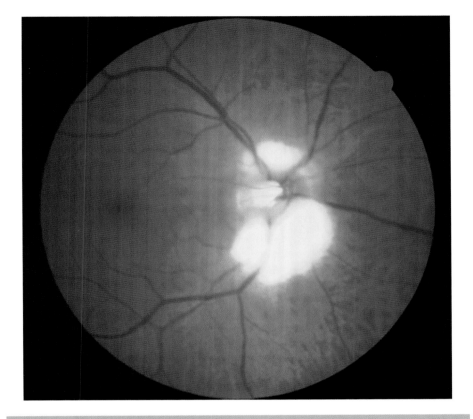

Figure 6.6 Myelinated fibres

Disc

The outline of the disc is over-shadowed and distorted by extensive pale areas. The appearance is that of a pale sheet extending from the optic disc for some distance but then gradually giving way to normal retina. The appearance of myelinated fibres is sometimes restricted to a narrow band stretching from the disc. The appearance is caused by a congenital variation in the nerve fibres which run across the retina. Most nerves elsewhere in the body have a myelin sheath, but this is normally not present in the retina. This normal variant carries no clinical significance.

Vessels

The vessels are obscured by the myelinated nerve fibres to a variable extent. The veins are moderately engorged although the vein running down from the disc appears irregular in outline just beyond the myelinated nerve fibres. This effect has been produced by the variation in light intensity in this area and was not present in the nasal view of the same eye.

Retina

Especially around the periphery of the image the retina shows pale bands separated by darker retina. This is a tiger-striped retina (see Figures 6.4 and 6.5). The variation in background colour makes careful examination of the retina difficult. The task is made easier on screen by changing the image view to 'red-free'. There are no retinal abnormalities on this image.

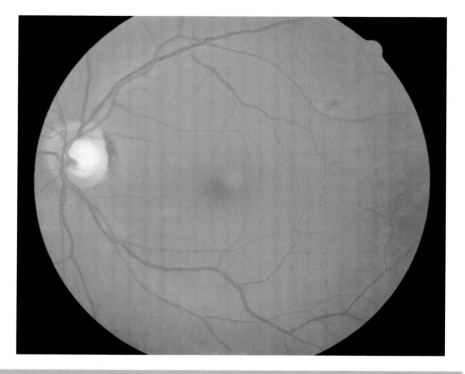

Figure 6.7 Myopic crescent

Disc

The margins are clearly visible, although the edge of the disc nearest the fovea is marked out with a thickened dark area. This is referred to as a myopic crescent, as it is most often seen in short-sighted eyes. The elongated eyeball is associated with the retina not entirely covering the choroid layer. The black choroid layer can thus be clearly seen. The appearance is entirely normal and results in no functional disturbance. The optic cup is around the upper limit of normal in size. The small vessels on the disc are normal.

Vessels

The vessels are unremarkable along their length.

Retina

A faint tiger-striped appearance can be made out especially peripherally. Careful examination segment by segment reveals a cluster of microaneurysms and haemorrhages lateral to and above the macular. This is associated with a cotton wool spot. There are several small hard exudates just above this area. Other microaneurysms are scattered in the lateral part of the image.

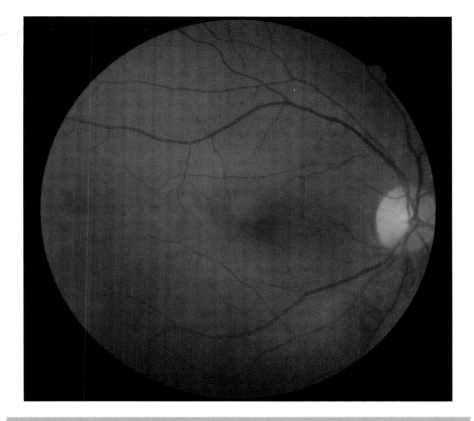

Figure 6.8 Pigmented image

Disc

The disc margins are very clearly delineated. A small optic cup is visible.

Vessels

The small vessels on the disc are single and normal. The veins are unremarkable.

Retina

The overall appearance of the retina is considerably darker in people with non-white skin. The intensity of flash has been turned up in order to ensure that the image is not too dark. There happens to be mild tiger-striping on this image. Just above the fovea is a pale area, and this is a reflection of the flash bulb. The pale area was absent on the corresponding disc centred film. In order to ensure that there are no diabetic changes it is important to view such dark films using digital lightening of the image.

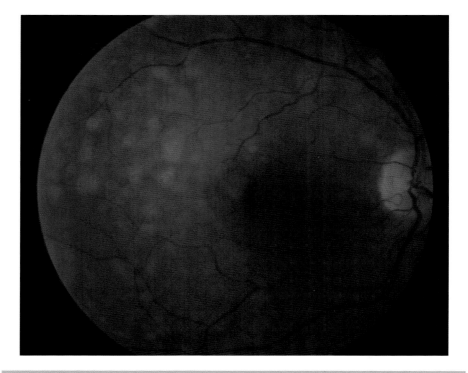

Figure 6.9   Asteroid hyalosis

Disc

The disc is unremarkable in outline. One small vessel takes a looped course before heading over the retina towards the fovea, but this is within normal. All other small vessels are single.

Vessels

The veins are moderately engorged. A single arteriole venous crossing change can be seen above the disc.

Retina

Examination of the retina segment by segment reveals the presence of numerous round pale spots of varying intensity. Visual acuity was normal in this eye. There had been no previous laser therapy. The appearance is a result of multiple small opacities in the vitreous humour each of which reflects the light of the flash. It is usually possible to obtain sufficient views of the retina in order to be able classify correctly any retinopathy present, but referral for slit lamp examination should be undertaken if there is any doubt about this. The image is dark, but can be manipulated on screen to allow examination.

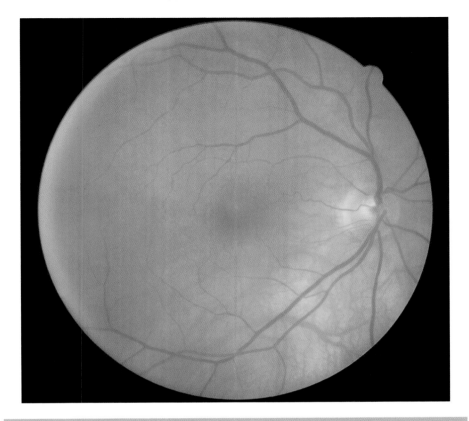

Figure 6.10 Choroidal circulation

Disc

The portion of the margin nearest the macula is defined but appears to have bal-
looned out from the expected curve. This is seen especially in short-sighted eyes (see
myopic crescent above). The relative pallor of the disc is normal in the context of
this relatively light image.

Vessels

The vessels are unremarkable.

Retina

Examination of the retina clockwise from just above the disc is normal until the area
towards the margin of the image below the disc is reached. Here the background
retina is pale and there appears to be a tangle of blood vessels which are less clearly
defined than usual. The appearance may raise concerns about new vessel formation.
However, it can be seen that the larger indistinct vessels are running as arcs across
the lower part of the image – the wrong direction for retinal vessels and too organized for new vessels. These vessels are part of the choroid circulation. They are most
often seen in the lower half of images but occasionally may be seen in the upper half
too.

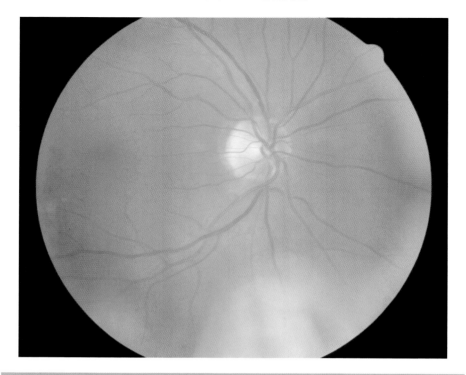

Figure 6.11   Eyelash artefact

Disc

The disc margins are clearly seen. Although the nasal half of the disc appears pinker than the temporal half the colour is even and there is no suggestion that this is abnormal. The small vessel running down at 6 o'clock to the centre of the disc requires careful inspection, but it is single and unremarkable. Similarly all the other small vessels on the disc are normal.

Vessels

There are stripes of light reflection along the length of many of the arterioles. The veins are normal but are made to look irregular in some areas due to light reflection, and these irregularities were not present in the macula centred view of the same eye.

Retina

Searching the retina in the usual fashion, the first notable feature is the right-hand margin of the image which is both darker and brighter. This is an edge artefact possibly caused by the edge of the iris being caught by the flash. The predominant feature of the image are the three pale fingers reaching in from the lower margin, coalescing and fading out further towards the centre of the image. The position and fairly clearly defined long edges make these typical of eyelashes which reflect the flash. Elsewhere on this image are two faint blot haemorrhages.

7

Background Retinopathy

What is background retinopathy?

Background retinopathy refers to the earliest visible changes in the retina due to diabetes. At this stage there is no imminent threat to sight although there is the clear implication that the person is susceptible to ongoing micro-vascular damage. Action is required to optimize blood pressure and blood glucose control.

Lesions

The three main lesions of background retinopathy are microaneurysms, blot haemorrhages and exudates.

Microaneurysms. These appear as small red dots on the retina. They are a result of ballooning of capillaries and are regarded as the earliest visible sign of diabetic retinopathy.

Blot haemorrhages. Rupture of small blood vessels in the deeper layers of the retina cause larger red lesions. They are approximately round but often with some irregularity of outline. The shape is determined by their position in the retina as they arise in the deeper layers where nerve fibres run perpendicular to the retinal surface. Although they look alarming to patients they do not cause functional disturbance.

Exudates. Leakage of plasma from capillaries causes yellow–white lesions with well-defined margins. Away from the macula region isolated exudates are not of particular concern. However, if they are within one disc diameter of the fovea the classification of the appearance changes from background to exudative maculopathy (see Chapter 9).

Cotton wool spots. When the capillaries in a small area of retina fail to deliver enough oxygen to the nerve fibres the area becomes pale with hazy, indistinct edges. This is due to swelling of the nerve fibres themselves. One or two cotton wool spots are not concerning, but if many are present referral is essential.

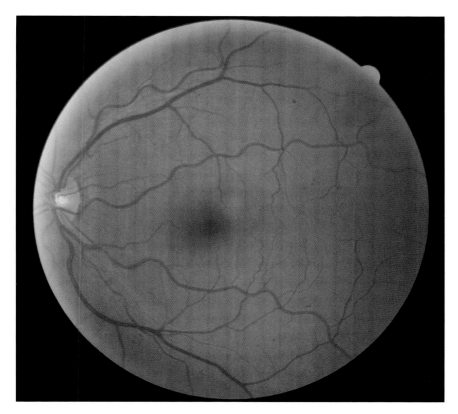

Figure 7.1 Early background

Disc

Normal colouring with unremarkable cup. Clearly defined temporal margin and less distinct but normal upper and lower margins.

Vessels

Veins are normal throughout with no abnormal variation in calibre. The ratio of vein to artery diameter is about 3:2.

Retina

Searching section by section from above the disc and moving in a clockwise direction, the first lesion encountered is a small, rather indistinct haemorrhage close to the edge of the image at 11 o'clock to the Fovea. Several microaneurysms are present between the uppermost vein and the artery below. Many other small red lesions are present. There are no lesions within one disc diameter of the fovea.

Early background retinopathy.

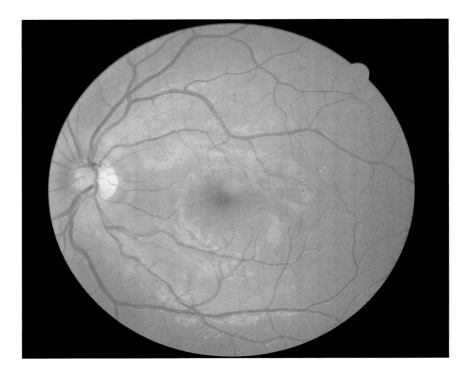

Figure 7.2   Early background

Disc

Unremarkable colour. Several small vessels present, but all single and running in purposeful directions.

Vessels

Veins of even calibre throughout even though the light reflection artefacts give an appearance of irregularity of the uppermost vein, about two and a half disc diameters from the disc. Light reflection is seen along the lower vein, linear for most of its length but intermittently broken in pattern. This is entirely normal.

Retina

Microaneurysms and small blot haemorrhages are encountered in the section just above the disc. Other red lesions are widely scattered elsewhere. There are two exudates several disc diameters lateral to the fovea. Note the difference in sharpness and shape between these and the flocculated pattern of light reflection nearer the centre. There is a small pale area at 2 o'clock to the fovea which is relatively poorly defined and has the same off-white colour as the light reflections. It was not visible on the disc centred image of this eye and was therefore confirmed as a reflection artefact.

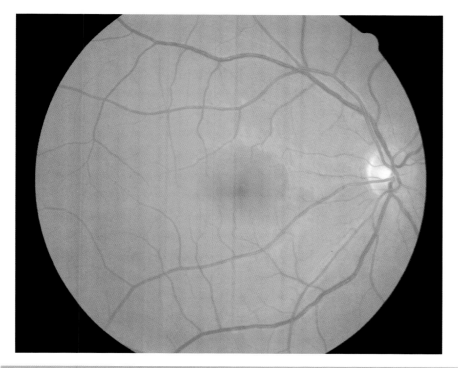

Figure 7.3 Early background

Disc

The disc is unremarkable.

Vessels

The vessels are normal throughout their length.

Retina

Examination of the image segment by segment reveals a few microaneurysms and small blot haemorrhages. Moving round the image clockwise from the disc the first two lesions are close together, immediately below the fovea and almost at the edge of the image. A micoaneurysm can be seen close to the arteriole which runs from the disc, below the macular region and branches right to the edge of the image. The microaneurysm is about one and a half disc diameters from the edge of the image. There is a small hard exudate just over one disc diameter above this. Following the arteriole running from the disc and above the macular region two microaneurysms can be seen below this, and one just above the arteriole. This image shows minimal background retinopathy. There is a faint light reflection artefact surrounding the macular region.

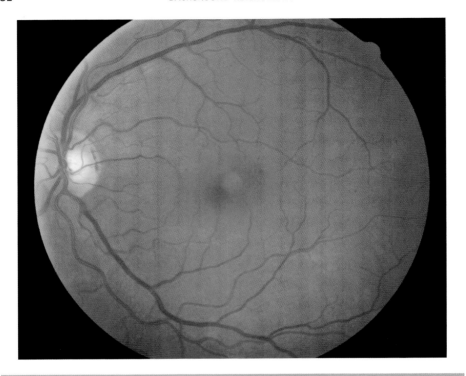

Figure 7.4   Early background

Disc

The visible portion of the disc shows normal margins, cup and small vessels. The appearance of a 'double margin' on the right-hand side of the disc is normal.

Vessels

The veins are engorged (ratio 2:1) but otherwise unremarkable throughout their length.

Retina

Working round the retina segment by segment at least 10 red lesions can be seen in the upper part of the film and at least six in the lower part of the film. There is a pale circle of reflection from the bulb just above the fovea. Three of the red lesions are within one disc diameter from the fovea, but visual acuity was better than 6/12 and so this film would not be reported as 'referable maculopathy'.

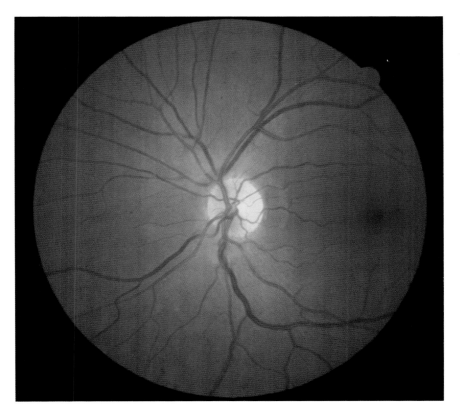

Figure 7.5   Early background

Disc

The disc is unremarkable, with normal variation of colour across its surface.

Vessels

The vessels are normal, although the arteries and veins twist round each other especially just below disc. The proximity of an artery and a vein at the edge of the image
and below the disc gives the initial appearance of variation in venous calibre, but
closer inspection shows the presence of two vessels.

Retina

Commencing with the segment above the disc, four microaneurysms and one haemorrhage can be seen in this sector alone. There is a blot haemorrhage half of a disc
diameter away from the fovea. Other haemorrhages and microaneurysms are scattered throughout the rest of the retina.

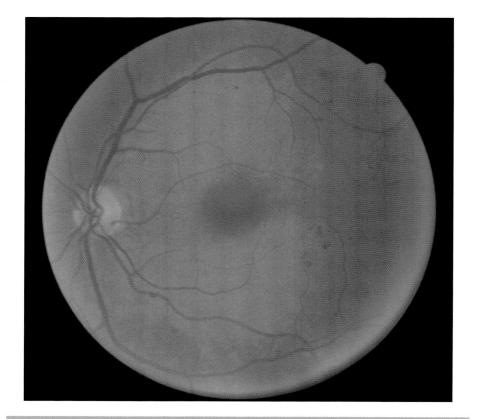

Figure 7.6   Moderate background

Disc

The colour, cup and vessels are normal.

Vessels

The upper vein is dilated, with a diameter at least twice that of the artery close by. Such dilatation is typical of marked hyperglycaemia. There is no irregularity of calibre. Arterio–venous nipping is present at several crossings.

Retina

Very many microaneurysms and blot haemorrhages are present. Do not let this distract you from the systematic search, section by section. There are several deep round haemorrhages. There are no indications for referral but full explanation to the patient of the appearance and its implication is necessary. Good control of blood pressure and blood glucose will slow the rate of progression.

8

Severe Non-proliferative ('Pre-proliferative') Retinopathy

Severe non-proliferative retinopathy refers to venous abnormalities (irregularity in calibre and looping) together with deep, round haemorrhages and widespread retinal abnormalities. Action is required to optimize blood pressure control and to refer to the ophthalmologist. Blood glucose control must not be acutely tightened as this is likely to cause rapid deterioration in the retinopathy.

Deep round haemorrhages.   These are larger and darker than blot haemorrhages, and indicate capillary fragility in the deeper layers of the retina.

IRMA.   Intraretinal microvascular anomalies are dilated small vessels which appear as small, squiggly vessels on the retina not obviously connected to veins or arteries.

Venous abnormalities.   Loops arising from veins and clear irregularities in the calibre of veins are the most important features suggesting imminent risk of proliferative change.

Handbook of Retinal Screening in Diabetes, Roy Taylor
© 2006 John Wiley & Sons, Ltd

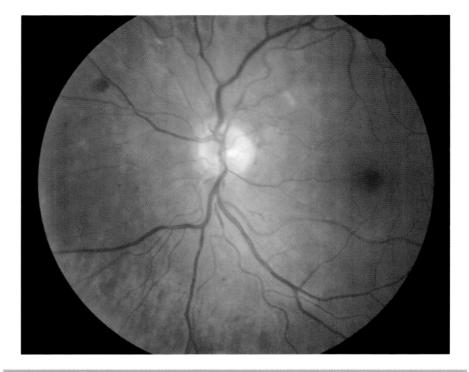

Figure 8.1 Severe non-proliferative retinopathy

Disc

Unremarkable.

Vessels

The vein at 12 o'clock to the disc is considerably dilated (the ratio of vein to arteriole diameters 3:1) and other veins are also dilated. The vein crossing the disc margin at 9 o'clock is irregular in calibre along its length.

Retina

At 1 o'clock to the disc there is a cotton wool spot. Below this there are several small squiggly vessels on the retina – these are IRMA. Microaneurysms and blot haemorrhages are scattered over the entire retina. There are some tiny exudates at the right-hand margin of the image. IRMA can be seen in several places, such as close to the very faint cotton wool spot at 7 o'clock to the disc, two thirds of the distance between disc and edge. There is one large, round haemorrhage. This is severe non-proliferative retinopathy and indicates the need for aggressive management of blood pressure and requires to be referred.

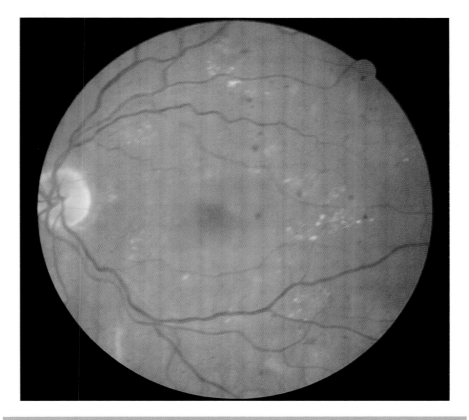

Figure 8.2 Severe non-proliferative retinopathy

Disc

Unremarkable.

Vessels

There is obvious irregularity in calibre of several veins, especially in the major vein of the inferior arcade.

Retina

The image has a slightly blurred appearance as a result of a central cataract. However, the vessels can be seen after the second branchings and the technical quality of this image is sufficient to indicate a very clear decision. Searching the retina as usual in a clockwise fashion from above the disc reveals multiple deep round haemorrhages, many exudates (including a circinate exudate at 12 o'clock to the fovea close to the edge of the image), and several cotton wool spots. Refer.

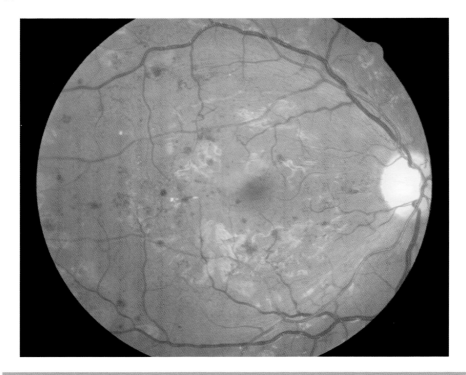

Figure 8.3   Severe non-proliferative retinopathy

Disc

A tiny vessel at 12 o'clock on the disc appears looped and in itself would justify further examination.

Vessels

The veins are engorged (ratio 2:1). There are arterio–venous crossing changes affecting the superior vein of the arcade. It is difficult to be sure that venous calibre is regular throughout because of the presence of marked changes on the surrounding retina in the lower half of the image. Following the veins to their disappearance in the upper half of the image leads the eye to venous loops and ragged extensions of veins.

Retina

There are numerous deep round haemorrhages, blots and microaneurysms. There are several groups of IRMA below, lateral to, and above the fovea. This is severe non-proliferative retinopathy (originally called pre-proliferative retinopathy). Refer (but full marks for spotting the laser scars near the lower temporal margin of the image which suggest that the ophthalmologist is already involved).

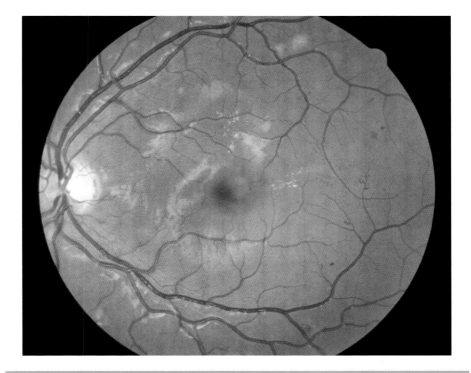

Figure 8.4 Severe non-proliferative

Disc

There is a small crescent of yellow at the temporal margin, and the vascular retina starts beyond this. The appearance is normal. The small vessels on the disc are all single and go in purposeful directions.

Vessels

Light reflection artefacts are prominent. The superior arcade of veins is normal. However, in following the branches of the inferior vein to their points of disappearance venous loops can be seen arising from the small veins in the temporal retina.

Retina

Small dilated vessels are scattered throughout the retina. There are patches of exudates just above and just lateral to the fovea. Compare the whiteness and shape of these with both the relatively featureless sheets of light reflection artefacts over the retinal surface and the hazy cotton wool spots near the edge of the upper temporal quadrant. Continuing the clockwise search of the retina, two longer abnormal vessels can be seen close to the larger cotton wool spot. These were reported to be IRMA by expert slit lamp examination, but are long enough to be regarded as possible new vessels and appear to arise from the vein. Refer.

9

Maculopathy

What is maculopathy?

The word simply means disease in the macular region of the retina. At the centre of the macula is the fovea, a tiny area responsible for all detailed vision and all colour vision. The rest of the retina is vast in comparison, but only provides low definition vision around the spot at which a person is looking. In practice, the brain 'fills in' the rest of the picture giving an illusion of detailed colour vision all round. Loss of vision at the fovea alone causes legal blindness. This is the commonest cause of blindness in diabetes. Detection of maculopathy is very important.

For the purposes of screening, the macula is defined as the area one disc diameter from the fovea. This definition allows a reasonably constant means of measuring distance inside the eye. Measurement with a ruler would not be useful because the image is magnified in different people to a different extent because of refractive differences. The optic disc of a short-sighted person will appear bigger than that of a normal or long-sighted person. The optic disc of a person who has had their lens removed and not artificially replaced will appear tiny. As all structures will be magnified to the same extent in any one image a relative measure is necessary.

Maculopathy is said to be present when there are any exudates, haemorrhages or microaneurysms in the macula region. This is a useful screening definition as it identifies all people at risk of losing foveal function. However, it must be understood that the visible signs of maculopathy are only indirect

Handbook of Retinal Screening in Diabetes, Roy Taylor
© 2006 John Wiley & Sons, Ltd

markers for the possible presence of macula oedema. It is the oedema which disrupts the fovea and causes loss of sight (see Chapter 3). Oedema, or swelling of the retina, cannot be seen on simple images. This is why ophthalmologists must use a slit lamp to allow stereoscopic assessment of whether the retina has become thickened.

Sight-threatening macula oedema does not occur without visible signs of retinopathy in the macula region. This means that an individual without visible maculopathy is most unlikely to be at risk of sight-threatening macula oedema. An individual with visible diabetic retinopathy in the macular region may or may not have macular oedema. For this reason many people referred with 'maculopathy' do not require laser therapy.

Theoretically, a drop in visual acuity (of two lines or more on the Snellen chart) could indicate the presence of macula oedema if there is no other explanation. In practice this would be exceptionally rare in the absence of visible maculopathy but as a doctrine of caution such a drop in visual acuity means that referral for slit lamp examination is required.

Management of maculopathy

A three-pronged attack is needed. Blood pressure control must be assured, blood glucose control must be as good as feasible for the individual, and referral to an ophthalmologist is required.

Blood pressure control

Exudation of plasma from the capillaries is increased if the pressure inside is too high. Both exudates and macula oedema will be affected directly by this physical factor even though the damage to the capillary wall may have taken years to develop. Referral to the doctor responsible for the patient's care is important so that blood pressure can be considered. If the systolic pressure (the higher number) is greater than 130 mmHg then treatment should be commenced. Treatment for hypertension is urgent and the usual two steps in blood pressure reduction may be postponed. Normally, salt in the diet will be advised to be decreased and weight loss, if necessary, will be emphasized. However, blood pressure tablets should be started without delay if maculopathy is associated with raised blood pressure. Up to five different types of blood pressure tablets may be needed for some people.

Blood glucose control

Referral to the doctor responsible for the patient's care is important so that blood glucose control can be considered. This is never a simple matter as many factors underlie just how low blood glucose levels should be (Chapters 1 and 2). Achievement of better blood glucose control will help slow down the progression of maculopathy and any associated macula oedema over the following months and years. It is important although less urgent than blood pressure control.

Referral to ophthalmologist

The ophthalmologist will perform slit lamp examination and assess whether sight-threatening macula oedema is present. If the ophthalmologist finds that there is no sight-threatening macula oedema, a decision will be taken whether to review in a few months, when laser treatment may become necessary, or whether to discharge back to the screening programme. Some visible exudates can be predicted to be unlikely to progress to serious disease in a short time.

If sight-threatening macula oedema is present then it is likely that grid laser therapy will be applied. This involves placing laser spots in a grid pattern just to the outer edge of the macula region of the affected eye. The mechanism of effect is not certain, but this has a good chance of decreasing the macula oedema and saving sight. However, unlike the almost complete success of laser therapy for proliferative disease, laser for macular oedema saves sight in only about 60 per cent of cases.

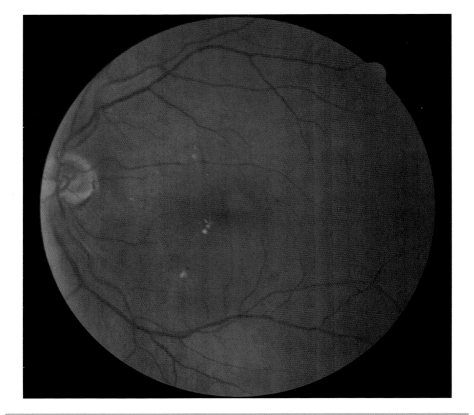

Figure 9.1   Exudates close to the fovea

Disc

There is variation in colour over the disc area and careful inspection of the disc-centred view would be necessary. The edge as seen is unremarkable. The darker linear pigmentation to the right and lower margins is a normal variant (myopic crescent).

Vessels

There appears to be A–V nipping just above the disc, although this is close to the disc and there are no other instances of this elsewhere. This is within normal limits rather than suggesting hypertension. The veins are of even calibre throughout.

Retina

Small blot haemorrhages are present in every segment of the retina. Hard exudates are present just to the right of the disc and within the arcades, below the fovea. The cluster of exudates just below the fovea are well within one disc diameter from the fovea. Refer.

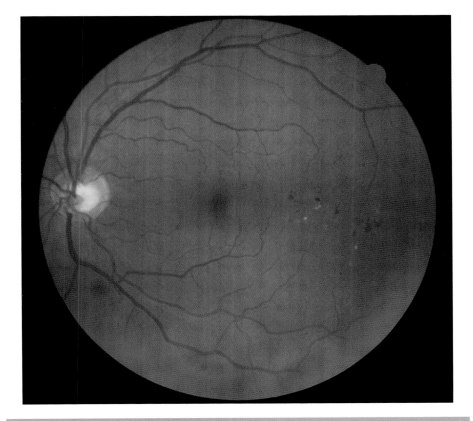

Figure 9.2 Severe retinopathy close to the macula

Disc

The optic cup is prominent although just less than 50 per cent of the disc diameter in size. The margins are very clear and normal.

Vessels

The veins are of even calibre with no abnormal features.

Retina

Microaneurysms are widely scattered. Blot haemorrhages and exudates are clustered lateral to the macula region. There is a larger resolving haemorrhage just over one disc diameter below the disc. The exudates are just over one disc diameter from the fovea but there are several red lesions within the critical zone. The fluffy, pale appearance at the lower edge of the image is likely to be an artefact relating to the lower eyelashes. This image does not strictly fall into the referable category, but it is most important that the need for aggressive blood pressure control is communicated to the doctor responsible for diabetes care.

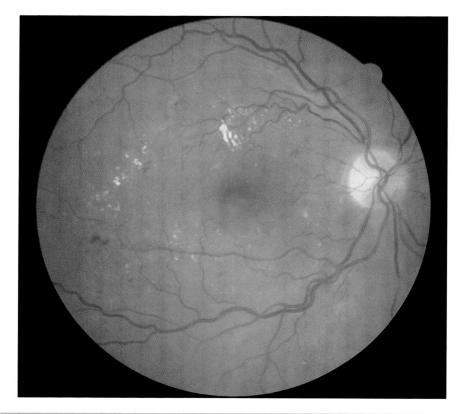

Figure 9.3 Widespread exudates

Disc

Unremarkable. Small vessels can clearly be seen to be single and having a definite direction.

Vessels

The veins are of normal calibre throughout. Note the curly path of some of the vessels which is a normal variant.

Retina

Many exudates are obvious between the arcades. One disc diameter above the fovea there is a suggestion of a circinate exudates, one part of which forms a confluent plaque of exudate. There are microaneurysms and blot haemorrhages all over the retina. Refer.

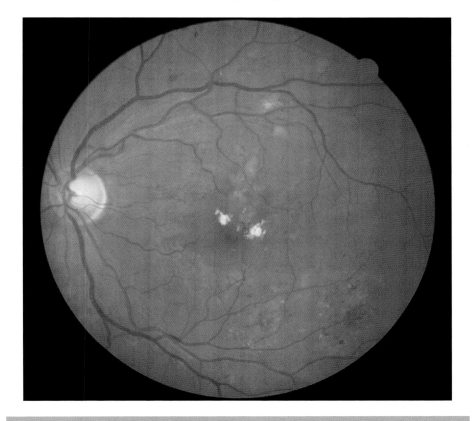

Figure 9.4 Large plaque exudates

Disc

Unremarkable, with a normal optic cup and normal small vessels.

Vessels

There are two arterio–venous crossing changes.

Retina

Starting from above the disc and moving clockwise, many microaneurysms and haemorrhages can be seen. There are a few exudates in the upper part of the image together with two cotton wool spots. The most obvious features are the large plaques of exudates with scattered smaller exudates very close to the fovea. In the lower part of the image close inspection is required to see that the red streaks are haemorrhages rather than IRMA. Such flame-shaped haemorrhages suggest hypertension, and the exudative maculopathy certainly requires attention to blood pressure by the doctor responsible for diabetes care. Refer.

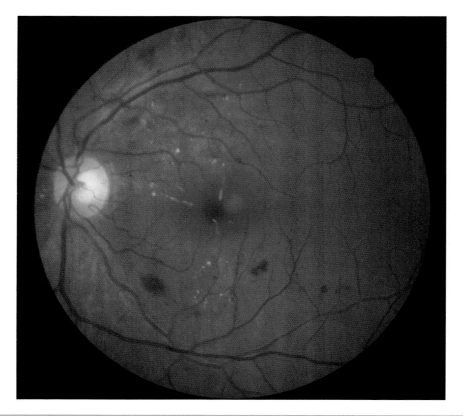

Figure 9.5   Linear exudates close to the fovea

Disc

The disc is pale with very clear margins and an optic cup which is about 50 per cent of the disc diameter. Although the possibility of this being a glaucomatous disc may be considered, the optic cup is just within normal size and the paths of the vessels are normal.

Vessels

Normal throughout.

Retina

There are several deep, round haemorrhages. Many exudates are present within the arcades. Note the linear configuration of the exudates close to the fovea which is likely to be a result of exudation in the nerve fibre layer where nerve fibre bundles are running away from the fovea. This macula star appearance is seen in hypertension although in this image there are no other features of hypertension. The variation of degree of pigmentation towards the lower margin of the image is normal. Refer.

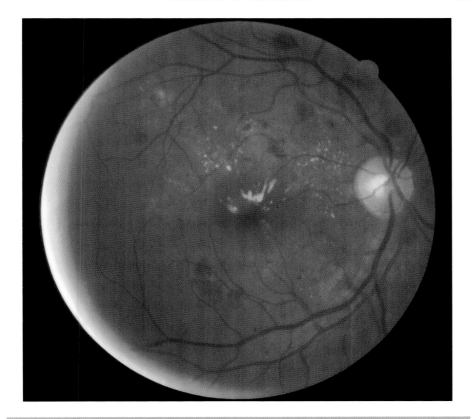

Figure 9.6   Plaque exudates near the fovea

The left eye partner of this image is shown in Figure 9.5.

Disc

The disc has normal colour, optic cup and margins.

Vessels

There is a hint of irregularity in calibre of the main vein towards the lower margin of the image.

Retina

The most important lesions are the exudates which are very close to the fovea and forming confluent plaques. Multiple exudates are present within the arcades. The multiple deep round haemorrhages suggest severe retinopathy. There is a cotton wool spot at 11 o'clock to the fovea, about three disc diameters away. Refer.

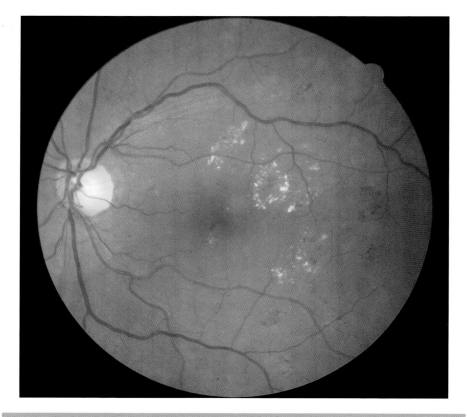

Figure 9.7   Circinate exudates within the arcades

Disc

A careful inspection is required to be sure that there are no abnormal vessels, but each of the smaller vessels can be seen to be single and purposeful.

Vessels

The veins vary somewhat in calibre. The vein above and to the right of the disc appears very irregular, but this is an optical consequence of intertwining with the adjacent artery.

Retina

The exudates are numerous and prominent. There is a circinate exudate which alone would dictate referral as it is within the arcades. It also comes within one disc diameter of the fovea. There are also single exudates close to the fovea. There are microaneurysms and blot haemorrhages throughout the image. Refer.

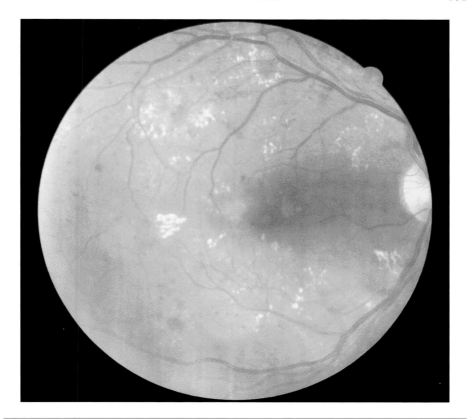

Figure 9.8   Widespread exudates with circinates

Disc

The disc cannot be judged from this image, which is not well centred on the macula.

Vessels

The vessels are unremarkable.

Retina

The macula region is not well seen despite the flash intensity having been increased to obtain this image of the eye of an Asian person. However, the image allows a clear interpretation. There are sheets of exudates, some of which are coalescing, in several areas on the retina. Several exudates can be seen close to the fovea. There are blot haemorrhages and a few microaneurysms. Flame-shaped haemorrhages can be seen near the vessels above the disc. The pale, ghost-like circular areas in the lower part of the image are light reflections from vitreous opacities (see Figure 6.9). Refer.

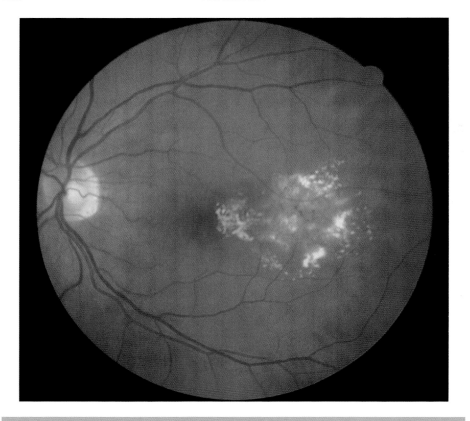

Figure 9.9   Coalescent exudates in the macula region

Disc

The lateral margin is clear and there are several small normal vessels. Note that the image is well centred, but as the retina appears magnified more than usual the whole disc is not included. This person must be short-sighted.

Vessels

Normal.

Retina

There are a few microaneurysms scattered in the periphery, but the major pathology is strikingly contained in the macula region. There is a coalescent arc of exudates which almost encircles the fovea. Multiple microaneurysms and blot haemorrhages can be seen within the central area. Refer.

10
Proliferative Retinopathy

What is proliferative retinopathy?

New vessels grow in an attempt to supply the retina with oxygen and food. They may arise from the disc or from the retina. Retinal new vessels often grow from veins, and for this reason veins need to be inspected along their length in all images. Proliferative retinopathy may occur without major background changes.

The new vessels are fragile and when they burst blood is released into the space in front of the retina. This is referred to as a pre-retinal haemorrhage. As the vitreous membrane has sometimes moved away from the retina, leaving a larger space, the haemorrhage may be both dense and extensive. Such a haemorrhage is referred to as a vitreous haemorrhage.

If blood glucose control is suddenly improved, proliferative retinopathy is made to progress more rapidly. Detection of proliferative retinopathy indicates the need for an urgent assessment of blood pressure control, and change in blood pressure management if necessary, as well as urgent referral to the ophthalmologist. All the images in this chapter should prompt referral.

Handbook of Retinal Screening in Diabetes, Roy Taylor
© 2006 John Wiley & Sons, Ltd

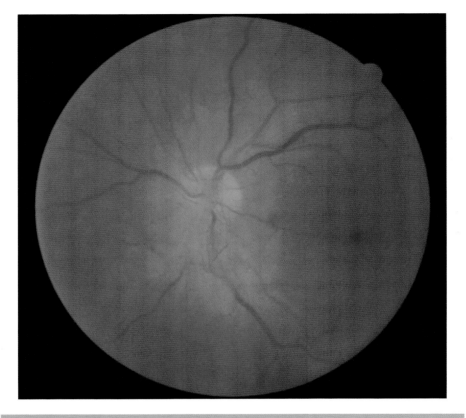

Figure 10.1   New vessels on the disc

Disc

The colour of the upper part of the disc is unremarkable, but the lower part looks blurred and pink. Close inspection shows a tangled mass of small fine vessels running both over the central part of the disc and inferiorly, obscuring the lower disc margin. The main vein running down from the disc is not clearly seen, and this is because the new vessels are growing along with a fibrous net of connective tissue.

Vessels

The veins are full, the vein:artery ratio of diameters being about 2:1. The vein running directly up from the disc is variable in calibre, and this can also be observed elsewhere. There are arterio–venous crossing changes.

Retina

Systematic examination of the rest of the retina shows relatively few other changes. The red lesions at 7 o'clock to the disc look like haemorrhages at first glance but they could be IRMA. In the context of the obvious new vessels this distinction is not important. One small haemorrhage is present at 10 o'clock to the disc. There are two long-standing naevi below the fovea.

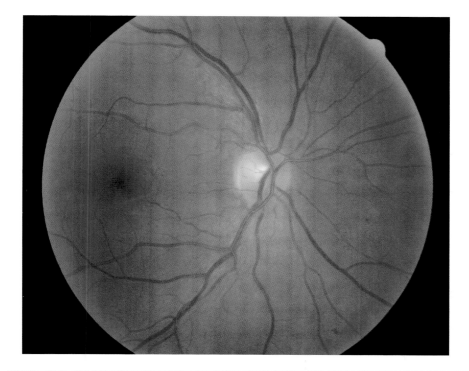

Figure 10.2   Disc new vessels

Disc

Following round the margin of the disc the small area of very fine vessels at 11 o'clock can be seen. This tangle of vessels extends upwards. Such fine new vessels could be missed if the systematic approach to each image is not followed.

Vessels

Apart from disc-associated new vessels the other blood vessels are unremarkable.

Retina

Microaneurysms and blot haemorrhages can be seen scattered throughout the retina. An IRMA is present close to one of the fine branches of an arteriole close to the margin of the image below the disk.

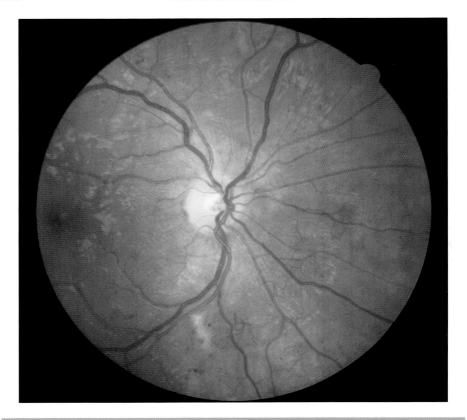

Figure 10.3   New vessels on the retina

Disc

The disc is normal colour with a well-defined cup. The margins are normal.

Vessels

The veins are engorged, with a 2:1 ratio compared to arteries. Following each from the disc to the edge of the image shows the upper vein to be moderately irregular in calibre. The vein at 3 o'clock to the disc flowers into a broad frond of fine new vessels. Just below this, a collection of spidery new vessels arise from the neighbouring vein. Further spidery new vessels overlie the artery running at 5 o'clock from the disc. A further collection of spidery new vessels arise from a vein at 6 o'clock to the disc.

Retina

The pattern of light reflection causes some difficulty in identifying exudates. There is a partial circinate exudate centred upon a red spot at 4 o'clock to the disc just beyond the new vessels. There is also a large plaque exudate at 6 o'clock to the disc close to several blot haemorrhages.

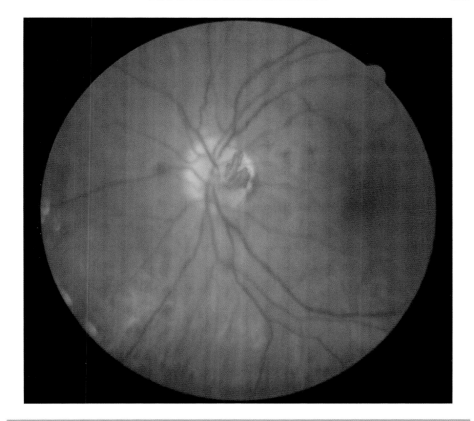

Figure 10.4 Disc new vessels

Disc

Obvious looped and irregular new vessels dominate the disc.

Vessels

Unremarkable as far as can be seen.

Retina

The image appears as though being viewed through bathroom glass, and this is due to the presence of cataract. The image is at the borderline of being interpretable for this reason, but this is irrelevant in view of the very clear abnormality demonstrated.

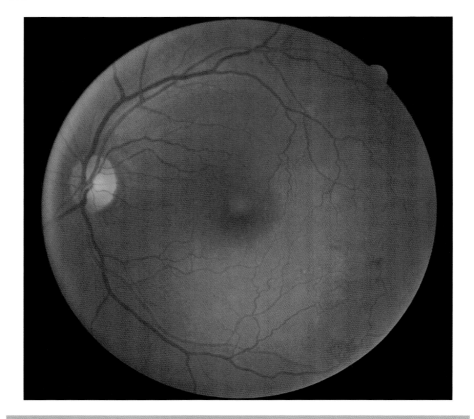

Figure 10.5 New vessels on the retina

Disc

The variation of colour over the disc is normal. The margins are well demarcated, and the slight irregularity of outline is often seen.

Vessels

The superior vein is engorged, with a ratio of almost 2:1 compared with the artery. The calibre of the vein varies and arterio–venous nipping is present. Following the superior vein to the end of each branch reveals no other abnormality.

The inferior vein is not obviously dilated, but does vary in calibre independently of the arterio–venous crossing changes. Following the vein out to the periphery leads the eye to two separate areas of fine, tangled new vessels.

Retina

There are three cotton wool spots in the upper half of the image. Microaneurysms and blot haemorrhages are scattered throughout. There is a patch of small exudates just above one of the areas of new vessels.

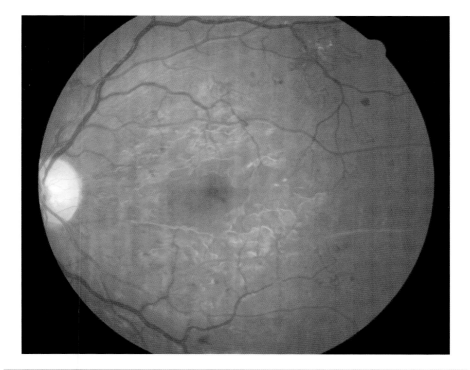

Figure 10.6 New vessels on the retina

Disc

The small vessels are not clearly abnormal.

Vessels

The veins are engorged. Following each out to the end of the branches leads the eye to a major tangle of new vessels in the upper temporal quadrant and a second tangle in the lower temporal quadrant. Careful inspection shows other areas of new vessels. There is an obstruction in one of the branches of the artery of the lower arcade, as seen by the ghost vessel. This is the distinct white line, complete with white branches, running towards the temporal edge of the image. It is difficult to judge whether some of the smaller veins in the lower part of the image are irregular because of the light reflection artefacts.

Retina

There are deep round haemorrhages, blots, microaneurysms and scattered exudates. The sheets of wavy white lines are light reflection artefacts, confirmed by their different appearance on the disc centred image of the same eye.

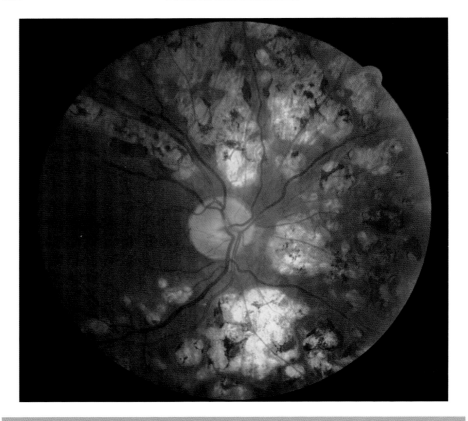

Figure 10.7 Old pan-retinal laser scars

Disc

A few tiny dilated vessels can be seen on the temporal side of the disc, these being the remnants of previous disc new vessels.

Vessels

The veins are irregular in calibre. This is especially so for the vein running down from the disc.

Retina

Above the disc is a large pale area with sharp edges. This is the scar left by several contiguous laser burns, and the pallor reflects destruction of capillaries in this area. The irregular red areas are haemorrhages which persist many years after laser therapy. Note that the pale scars do not involve the major vessels (unlike areas of old chorioretinitis) but rather fit between the vessels. Towards the upper margin of the image the choroidal circulation can be seen through the thinned retina. The irregular very dark blotches are exposed choroids, and such an appearance is common in association with laser scars. This is particularly so for older laser scars, as the more modern application of laser treatment does not apply such intense burns.

Although the image may look alarming, vision in this eye was 6/06 and the appearances have been stable for many years.

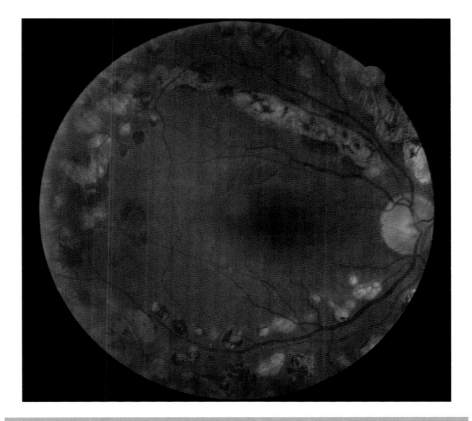

Figure 10.8 Pan-retinal laser scars

Disc

This image corresponds to the disc centred image in Figure 10.6. The tiny dilated vessels on the temporal side of the disc can be seen more clearly. These are the remnants of previous disc new vessels.

Vessels

Venous irregularity can be seen in both larger and smaller veins. One of the small branches of the inferior vein leads to an area of tangled new vessels. If observed as a development since last screening these would trigger referral, but in fact the appearance of this image had been stable for many years.

Retina

The laser burns can be seen to have been positioned along the main vessels of the arcade. The area between fovea and disc is never lasered. The scars are of different size and shape and some are confluent. Black choroids are exposed irregularly. A few superficial retinal haemorrhages can be seen towards the temporal side of the image. Some scattered microaneurysms are present.

11

Advanced Diabetic Eye Disease

What is advanced?

It is useful to group together retinal appearances which represent the late complications of retinopathy. Pre-retinal, vitreous, haemorrhages represent bleeding most often from new vessels. New vessel growth is accompanied by growth of a fibrous matrix, and this may persist after laser therapy. Steady contraction of this fibrous tissue over years may pull on the retinal and lead to retinal detachment. Even after successful laser treatment, the stimulation for new vessel growth may persist and the term rubeosis iridis refers to the involvement of the iris with major risk of acute (rubeotic) glaucoma.

All the images in this chapter would warrant immediate referral with the exception of those appearances already assessed by the ophthalmologist and known to be stable.

Handbook of Retinal Screening in Diabetes, Roy Taylor
© 2006 John Wiley & Sons, Ltd

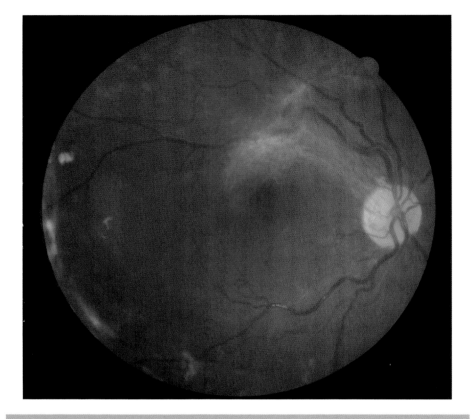

Figure 11.1   Early fibrosis

Disc

Several small tortuous vessels are present towards the temporal side.

Vessels

There is some variation in venous calibre. A venous loop arises from the inferior vein and small tangled new vessels can be seen arising from the other branches.

Retina

Arising from the disc there is a pale area of fibrosis. This extends upwards and it can be seen that the nearby veins appear distorted. A few IRMA can be seen in the vicinity of the temporal fibrous band. Above the superior arcade laser scars are present.

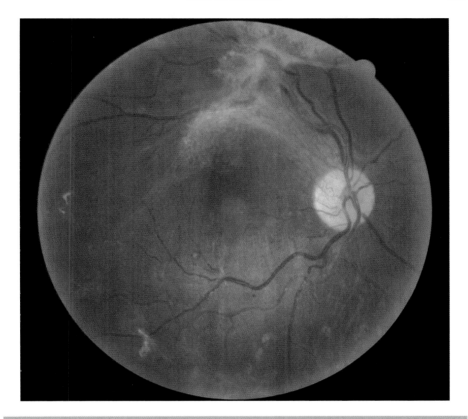

Figure 11.2 Fibrosis

This image was taken 1 year later from the eye shown in Figure 11.1. Compare these two images to observe how the vessels have become further distorted.

Disc

The small vessels running temporally on the disc remain tortuous.

Vessels

The traction effect of the fibrotic process is particularly obvious for the vein forming the superior arcade. Now the band of fibrous tissue extending upward is thicker. The small venous loop remains unchanged one disc diameter below the fovea.

Retina

The laser scars are still visible although fine retinal detail is not well seen. Vision in this eye is maintained at 6/09. However, continuing ophthalmological follow-up is required to determine when vitrectomy may be required to remove the fibrous bands and prevent further distortion.

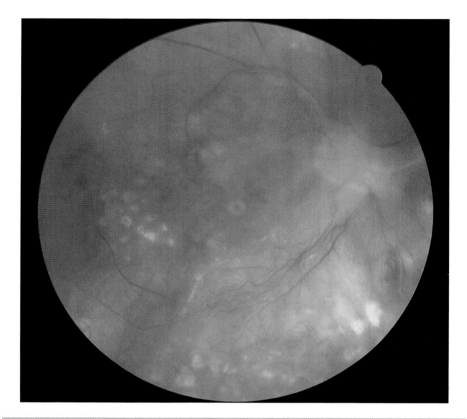

Figure 11.3   Fibro-vascular membrane

Disc

The disc is largely hidden by a fibrous sheet. This gives the appearance of blurring the disc margin, but the fibrous bands which radiate out are characteristic.

Vessels

The major vessels near the disc are obscured by the fibrous change. The main sheet of connective tissue runs diagonally down from the disc and contains two leashes of new vessels, one running diagonally and the other downwards.

Retina

Some laser scars are present below and temporal to the fovea and in the lower part of the image. Blot haemorrhages are present. The vision in this eye was 6/09.

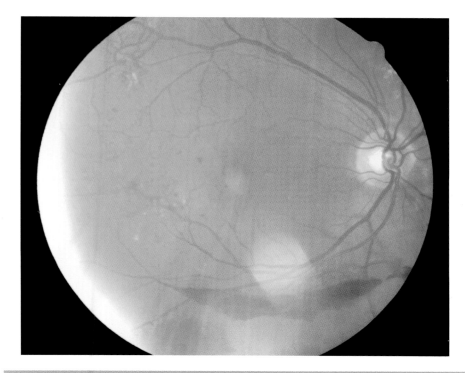

Figure 11.4 Pre-retinal haemorrhage

Disc

The disc is normal with a well-defined optic cup.

Vessels

Venous engorgement is present (ratio 3:1). Following the veins leads the eye to two separate tangles of new vessels.

Retina

The obvious haemorrhage is extensive and has relatively clearly defined borders. This has to be pre-retinal. The upper border is relatively horizontal, representing settling of the red blood cells under gravity. There are scattered exudates including in the macula region. The pale stripe with well-defined edges (lower edge of the image) is caused by the flash reflecting from an eyelash.

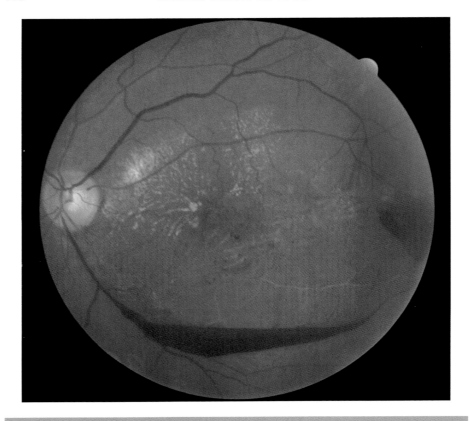

Figure 11.5   Pre-retinal haemorrhage

Disc
The disc is unremarkable with normal vessels, margins and cup.

Vessels
The veins are engorged, particularly in the upper half of the image where the ratio of vein to artery diameter is greater than 3 : 1 (normal 3 : 2). Near the temporal margin of the image there are some spidery new vessels. There may be some indistinct new vessels arising from the inferior temporal vein just over one disc diameter from the disc. The artery running down from the disc appears to become indistinct and can then seen to replaced by white lines running across the image. This indicates a complete and long-standing blockage of the artery.

Retina
Extensive hard exudates are present across the macula region and beyond. Microaneurysms and blot haemorrhages are seen below the fovea. The most obvious abnormality is a dark shape with a straight upper border across the lower part of the image. This is a pre-retinal haemorrhage. Blood has leaked into the space between the retina and the vitreous. The blood cells settle under gravity, causing the characteristic straight upper border. There is also an extensive haemorrhage near the temporal margin of the image which may represent a very recent pre-retinal haemorrhage as the upper border has not yet become distinct. It is most important that urgent referral to the doctor responsible for the diabetes care is organized to ensure that aggressive blood pressure control is in place. Urgent ophthalmological referral is also required.

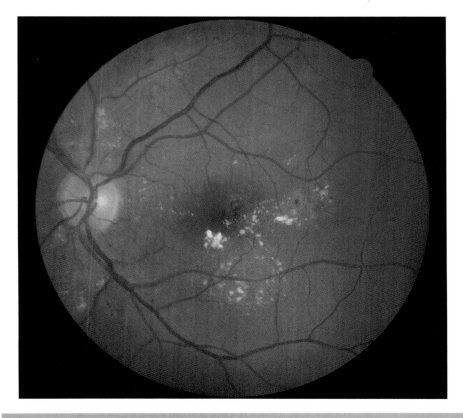

Figure 11.6 Severe exudative maculopathy

Disc

The disc is indistinct for much of its area, and it is impossible to exclude the presence of abnormal fine vessels, especially just beyond the margin of the disc at 6 o'clock.

Vessels

The vessels are unremarkable.

Retina

There are extensive sheets of exudates involving most of the retina. In several areas the exudates can be seen to be in an approximate circinate pattern. There is a large plaque of exudates encroaching on the fovea. A few small blot haemorrhages and microaneurysms are also present. Visual acuity was 6/60, reflecting macular oedema. Laser therapy is unlikely to be of benefit at this stage. Referral is still indicated.

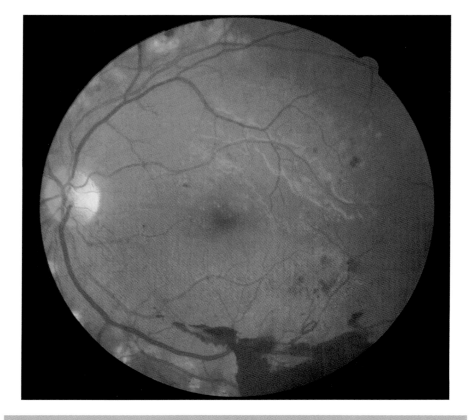

Figure 11.7   Pre-retinal haemorrhage and persisting new vessel formation

Disc

The disc margins are normal. Several normal small vessels are present in the upper portion of the disc. However, a tangle of small vessels leave the disc at around 5 o'clock, and these vessels form loops over the nearby retina.

Vessels

The calibre of the veins vary. The veins lead to several spidery new vessels in the lower part of the image. There is a pre-retinal haemorrhage in this region.

Retina

Laser scars are present above the disc. There are some scattered hard exudates in the macular region, although the linear streaks of white are in fact reflection artefacts. Several isolated, spidery new vessels can be seen.

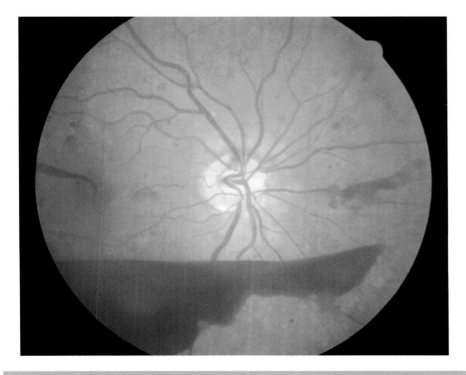

Figure 11.8 Pre-retinal haemorrhages

Disc

The disc margins are unremarkable. There is an indistinct red area over the upper and left-hand part of the disc. This is fibro-vascular tissue resulting from previous new vessel formation.

Vessels

The veins are engorged. There is some variation in calibre of the veins.

Retina

Multiple blot haemorrhages are present. At 3 o'clock to the disc there is a moderate sized pre-retinal haemorrhage. Below the disc there is a large pre-retinal haemorrhage which must have been present for sometime given that the blood cells have settled under gravity to cause the straight upper border. Some small dilated vessels can be seen towards the left-hand side of the disc, and are likely to be IRMA. A third pre-retinal haemorrhage extends over the macular region. Microaneurysms and more blot haemorrhages are present in the upper left-hand portion of the image.

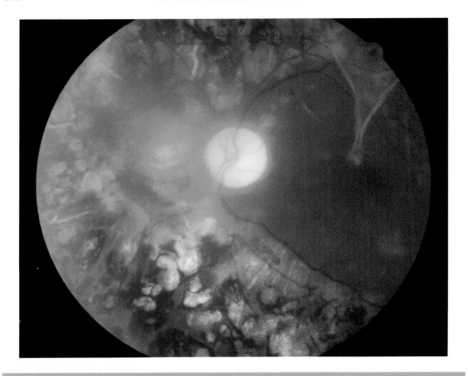

Figure 11.9   Fibrous band and heavy laser scars

Disc

The disc is unusually pale, probably as a result of poor microvascular circulation at the nerve head.

Vessels

The major vessels are poorly seen, being partially obscured by fibrous tissue extending forwards from the plane of the retina.

Retina

The distinct white band of fibrous tissue is attached to a small area of the retina near the fovea. Further contraction could cause distortion then detachment of the retina with catastrophic results upon the visual acuity of this eye. Visual acuity has been preserved by the photocoagulation over 10 years earlier (6/09) despite peripheral field defects. The very heavy laser therapy was necessary to halt the proliferative process which continued after standard pan-retinal photocoagulation.

12

Non-diabetic Eye Disease

What other diseases are common?

Many disease processes can affect the retina, often without causing symptoms.

Drusen spots are not uncommon in older people. They are caused by local degenerative changes in the structure of the retina but do not threaten sight. It is most important that the retinal screener is able to identify these confidently as unremarkable and not to diagnose mistakenly exudates. Otherwise excessive referrals to the ophthalmologist would occur.

Chorioretinitis caused by such past infections as toxoplasmosis can produce alarming signs which are of no current significance.

Hypertensive retinopathy is important to identify because the raised blood pressure is readily treated and such treatment can prevent strokes and other vascular diseases.

Papilloedema can indicate serious intracranial disease and full hospital investigation is required.

Naevi (moles) occur in the retina as often as they do on the skin. They require expert assessment unless they have previously been known to be present and show no change compared with previous images. The concern is that the dark spot is a malignant melanoma requiring urgent ophthalmological assessment and treatment.

Congenital retinal disorders may be seen and retinitis pigmentosa is most frequently encountered. People with this familial progressive disease will usually already be under ophthalmological care.

Central and branch vein retinal occlusions require ophthalmological assessment. Cholesterol emboli are likely to be associated with high blood cholesterol levels, and simple tablet treatment saves lives.

Other eye diseases

Glaucoma

Two very different diseases can cause raised pressure in the eyeball and they are often confused.

Chronic glaucoma (also known as open angle glaucoma) is common and by itself is the third commonest cause of blindness registration in the UK. It is caused by relative blockage of the outflow of aqueous humour through the trabecula meshwork into the canal of Schlemm. Chronic glaucoma is very gradual in onset and can cause substantial loss of vision before it is diagnosed. The optic disc may have an abnormally large cup. Older people are mainly affected, and 10 per cent of relatives are likely to develop the condition. Treatment is usually by the use of eye drops (e.g. timolol, latanoprost). Tropicamide eye drops do not constitute any risk for people with chronic glaucoma or their family members. Use of mydriatic drops is irrelevant to the cause of this condition.

Acute glaucoma (also known as angle closure glaucoma) is much less common and has less of a family tendency. It presents acutely as a painful, red eye and urgent ophthalmological treatment is essential. Predisposed people have a narrow angle between the cornea and the iris (see Figure 3.1) and sudden blockage of drainage to the canal of Schlemm can happen at any time. Treatment is by laser or surgery to create a hole in the iris, and this is done in both eyes. Once this has been done there is no risk of recurrence and mydriatic eye drops of any kind may be used. The great cloud of worry about this subject has been created entirely because people who are just about to develop acute glaucoma may have the condition precipitated by use of strong or combined mydriatic drops (such as atropine, cyclopentolate). This is a rare event. Even for such people in the days before they suffer the acute attack, the relatively weak tropicamide is extremely unlikely to precipitate acute glaucoma when used as a single agent.

Conjunctivitis

Inflammation of the conjunctiva is most often due to infection. Allergy or physical irritation may also cause a similar appearance. Viral conjunctivitis is very contagious and strict hygiene must be observed for any red eye. Expert diagnosis is necessary.

Sub-conjunctival haemorrhage

A minor leak of blood under the conjunctiva can cause an alarming appearance of uniform redness where there should be white conjunctiva. It may involve the whole or only part of the conjunctival area, and usually only affects one eye. Often no cause can be found, but it is typically associated with a bad coughing bout. A sub-conjunctival haemorrhage always gets completely better with no treatment and is of no concern whatever.

Uveitis

Uveitis is an inflammatory condition of the ciliary body and iris. It tends to be associated with systemic diseases such as inflammatory arthritis (e.g. ankylosing sponylitis, Reiter's syndrome, systemic lupus).

Box 12.1   Glaucoma

Chronic glaucoma

Due to slow drainage of aqueous humour from the eye even though the angle between the iris and the pupil is normal.

   Also known as open-angle glaucoma (and is unaffected by mydriatic drops).

   This is the common form of glaucoma.

   Tends to run in families.

Acute glaucoma

Due to blockage of drainage of aqueous humour from the eye because of closure of a narrower than normal angle between the iris and the pupil.

   Comes on suddenly with pain and redness of eye.

   In susceptible people it can be precipitated by strong mydriatic drops such as those used by ophthalmologists.

   It cannot be precipitated by tropicamide (0.5 or 1 per cent) unless spontaneous acute glaucoma was just about to happen anyway.

Treatment

Chronic glaucoma is usually treated with regular eye drops (such as timolol). Such treatment is not a contraindication to the use of tropicamide.

   Acute glaucoma is usually treated by creating a drainage hole through the iris either by laser or by surgery. Both eyes are treated, and after such treatment there is no contraindication to the use of tropicamide.

   The myth that tropicamide eye drops cannot be used in people with established glaucoma is simply without basis. The myth has created a real risk to eyesight by causing failure to screen properly for diabetic retinopathy.

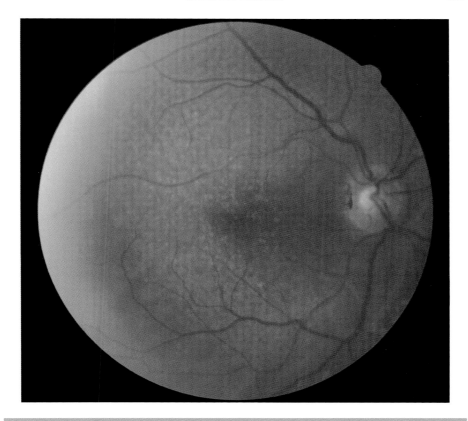

Figure 12.1   Drusen

Disc

The optic cup is well-defined and normal. Colour elsewhere on the disc is normal apart from a small linear haemorrhage. The disc margins are not clear but are within normal appearances.

Vessels

Normal.

Retina

Small, approximately round lesions are evenly spread over the central retina. Each is slightly indistinct and pale but not white. The most diagnostic feature of Drusen spots is that they are fairly uniformly distributed in most cases, as opposed to the random occurrence or clustering of exudates. If the white lesions are as obviously close to the fovea as in this case and the visual acuity is normal, the lesions are unlikely to be exudates.

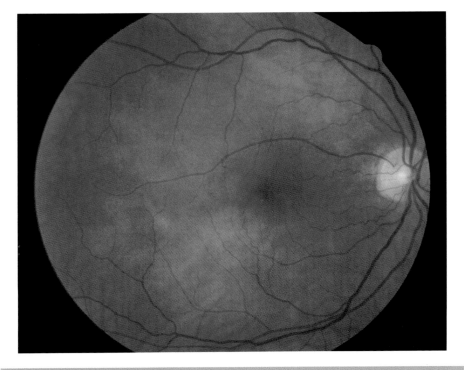

Figure 12.2   Drusen

Disc

Unremarkable, with normal cup, margins and small vessels.

Vessels

Normal.

Retina

Examination of the peripheral retina is unremarkable, with normal variation of background colour. Close to the fovea there are several pale areas, most of which are indistinct. One appears more prominent. Visual acuity was normal, and because a confident diagnosis could not be made ophthalmology referral was arranged. All lesions were confirmed as Drusen spots.

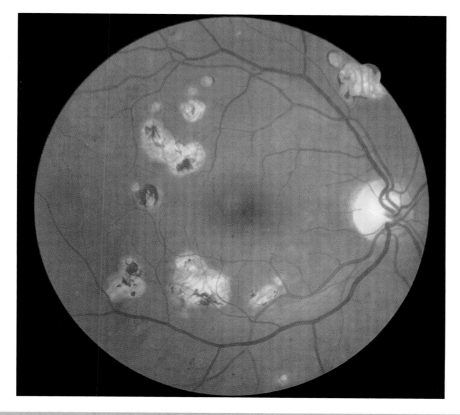

Figure 12.3   Atrophic chorioretinital scars

Disc

The colour, margins and small vessels are unremarkable.

Vessels

The veins are normal throughout with some light reflection especially in the lower part of the image. The diameter is somewhat greater than normal, approaching 3:2 compared with arteries.

Retina

Several very pale, well demarcated lesions are scattered over the retina. The shape varies, and some contain dark areas of pigment clumping. The retinal vessels frequently run across the lesions. The patient reported no previous eye trouble or serious illness and vision was perfect. The appearance of focal inflammation from many years ago can be expected to remain stable. There are also widespread microaneurysms and blot haemorrhages. The two small round pale spots in the macula region (one at 4 o'clock and one at 8 o'clock to the fovea) deserve comment. They look too regular and too tiny to be exudates. They are tiny intra-retina cysts.

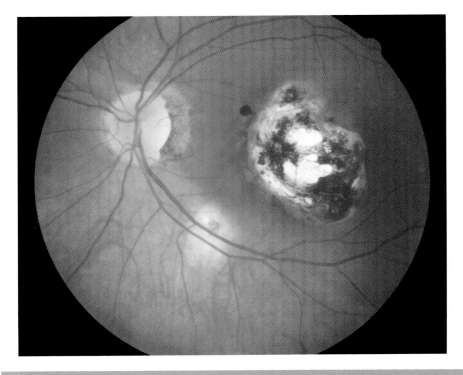

Figure 12.4   Old chorioretinitis

Disc

The disc is more oval shaped than usual and appears to have a raised right-hand margin. This is known as a tilted disc.

Vessels

The retinal vessels are unremarkable.

Retina

A large irregular scar on the retina replaces much retinal tissue. A second, less dramatic lesion is also present at 5 o'clock to the disc. There was a history of childhood toxoplasmosis (a worm infection carried by cats and dogs).

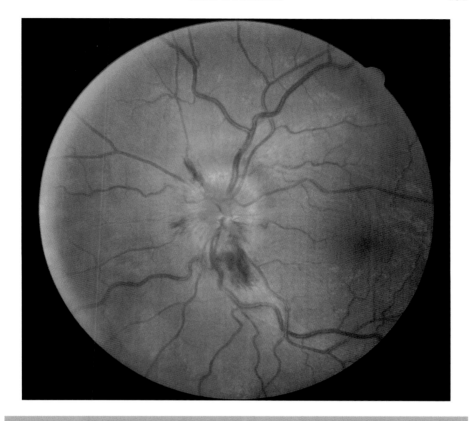

Figure 12.5 Papilloedema

Disc

The disc margin cannot be seen at all and the disc is strikingly pink. The cup is completely obliterated and the vessels appear to run across the disc before disappearing centrally.

Vessels

The veins are engorged throughout.

Retina

Flame-shaped haemorrhages are present radiating from the disc. Elsewhere the retina is unremarkable. Refer to a physician to diagnose the cause of the papilloedema.

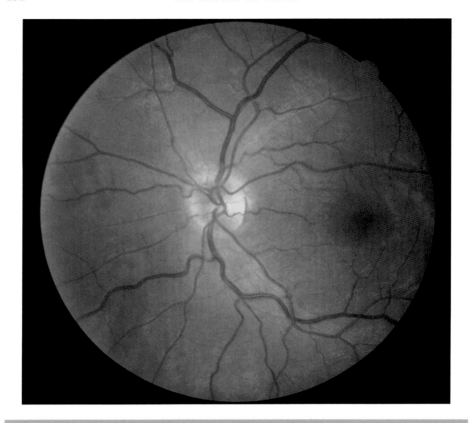

Figure 12.6   One year later – same eye as Figure 12.5

The papilloedema shown in Figure 12.5 was due to sleep apnoea, a treatable condition.

Disc

The disc has returned to normal colour – pale centrally and temporally with a pink tinge nasally. The temporal margin of the disc is now clearly defined. The nasal margin is rather indistinct but this is well within the range of normality.

Vessels

The veins remain wider than normal but they are not so engorged at the margins of the disc.

Retina

The flame-shaped haemorrhages close to the disc have completely resolved. The small blot haemorrhage has also disappeared. Some darkish pigmentation – tiger striping – is evident near the nasal edge of the image.

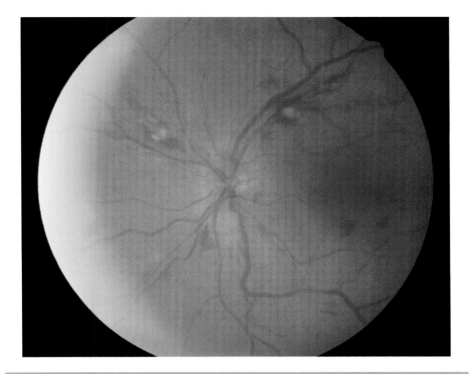

Figure 12.7   Papilloedema

Disc

The disc's margins are indistinct and the vessels run over the disc to disappear centrally. The disc is much pinker than usual.

Vessels

The veins are engorged. There are some arterio–venous crossing changes.

Retina

There are many flame-shaped haemorrhages over the whole retinal surface in keeping with the severe hypertension which was the cause of the papilloedema. Refer such an appearance to a physician to diagnose the condition underlying the papilloedema.

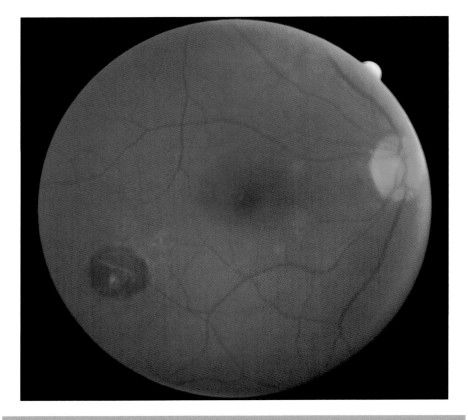

Figure 12.8   Pigment epithelial hypertrophy

Disc

The disc is partially seen but appears normal.

Vessels

The vessels are unremarkable along their lengths. Although the image is adequate to report, there is a faint 'ground glass' appearance which is a result of the presence of a moderate cataract.

Retina

There are some pale areas inside the arcades which have fairly indistinct margins and are palish rather than white. They are Drusen spots. The most obvious change is that of the darkly pigmented, almost circular lesion. It has as irregular margin and is crossed by blood vessels (which reflect light brightly against the black background). This well-defined lesion is clearly a naevus, and malignant melanoma must be excluded by referral to the ophthalmologist.

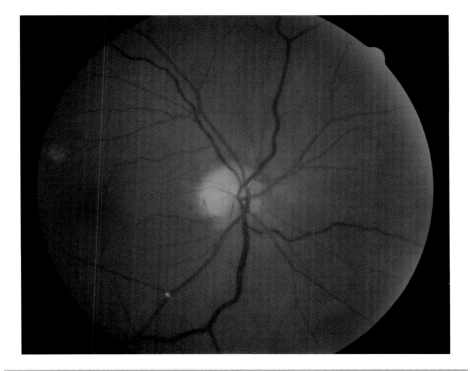

Figure 12.9 Cholesterol embolus

Disc

The nasal part of the disc is not clearly defined but there are no suspicious features. There is a dark area at the temporal edge of the disc which may be mistaken for a haemorrhage, but is a small area of visible choroid.

Vessels

The veins are normal, with normal tortuosity. There is a strikingly bright reflection of light at the first major branch of the inferior temporal artery. This is a cholesterol embolus, characterized by its brightness, and its position entirely within the artery at a branch point.

Retina

The diffuse pale area above and lateral to the fovea is a Drusen spot, and this diagnosis was made easier by the presence of others on the macula view of the same eye. There are two small round pale dots at 3 and 8 o'clock to the disc. Slit lamp examination showed these to be unremarkable retinal cysts.

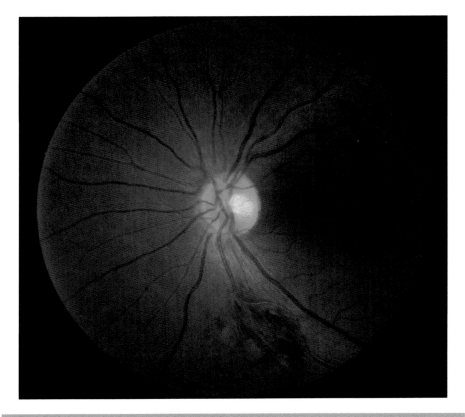

Figure 12.10   Branch retinal vein occlusion

Disc

Unremarkable.

Vessels

Unremarkable.

Retina

The image is rather dark, but digital lightening shows there to be no retinal lesions other than the obvious cluster of flame haemorrhages at 6 o'clock to the disc. The occurrence of lesions tightly grouped in one area with an otherwise normal retina makes it likely that this is caused by occlusion of the branch of one retinal vein. Refer to the ophthalmologist.

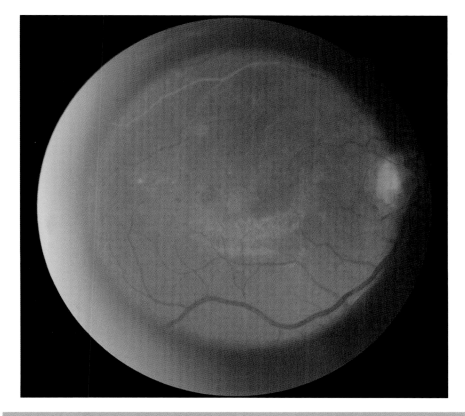

Figure 12.11 Branch retinal artery occlusion

Disc

Inadequately seen on this restricted view image.

Vessels

The vein of the lower arcade appears normal. The arteries in the upper arcade are mostly replaced by white lines. This indicates an arterial occlusion probably by thrombus, and blood is prevented from flowing into these sections.

Retina

Blot haemorrhages and exudates are present. Refer to the doctor in charge of the patient's diabetes as the overall vascular risk must be assessed. If there is any doubt about the diagnosis, refer to the ophthalmologist.

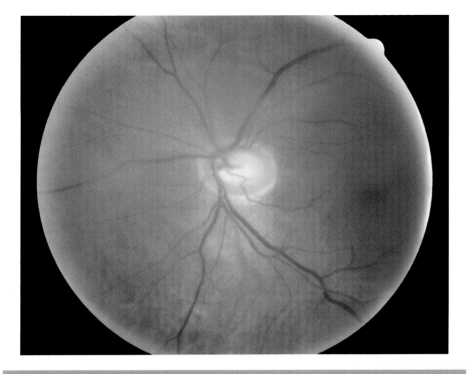

Figure 12.12   Glaucomatous disc

Disc

The large optic cup is immediately striking. It occupies more than 50 per cent of the disc diameter. The vessels running across the disc appear to roll down into the cup and can be seen running across the base of the cup itself.

Vessels

Unremarkable.

Retina

Unremarkable. Refer to the ophthalmologist (or optometrist depending upon local practice) for further examination.

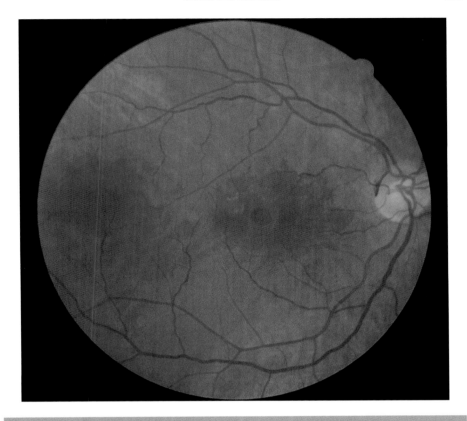

Figure 12.13   Macular hole

Disc

Normal cup, vessels and margins. There is a myopic crescent.

Vessels

Normal

Retina

Section by section examination of the retina shows no abnormalities outside the macular area. There is a red, very well demarcated patch close to the fovea. This is known as a macular hole, a limited tear of the retina in the region of the fovea resulting most often from a degenerating vitreous causing traction. It can cause significant loss of central vision. There are also a few exudates in the macula region. The dark shadow involving the macula is a photographic artefact due to relatively low flash intensity. Refer to the ophthalmologist for diagnosis and treatment.

Self-assessment Questions

For each topic indicate which of the five statements are correct and which are not.

Chapter 1

Type 1 diabetes:

(a) is caused by complete failure of the alpha cells of the pancreas

(b) has a peak age of onset around 13 years

(c) has a strong tendency to run in families

(d) affects approximately 0.3 per cent of the UK population

(e) is caused by an autoimmune destruction of insulin producing cells

At the time of diagnosis of type 1 diabetes:

(a) weight loss is typically present

(b) tiredness and passing excessive urine have usually been present for over a year

(c) it is never associated with skin complications

(d) there are usually ketones present in urine

(e) immediate treatment with insulin is vital

Handbook of Retinal Screening in Diabetes, Roy Taylor
© 2006 John Wiley & Sons, Ltd

For treatment of type 1 diabetes, insulin:

(a) is given by injection into muscle

(b) replaces a hormone which can no longer be made

(c) is supplied in different forms with different duration of action

(d) may be given as short-acting and intermediate-acting injections twice daily

(e) given as pre-meal short-acting insulin with a long-acting background injection can give better day-to-day flexibility

Eating in type 1 diabetes:

(a) is based around carbohydrate restriction

(b) must be preceded by weighing the food

(c) carbohydrate is estimated in 10 g portions

(d) a large potato is one 10 g portion

(e) sugar is a form of carbohydrate

Hypoglycaemia:

(a) may cause mental confusion, sweating and shakiness

(b) unconsciousness only occurs if the early warning signs are ignored

(c) is treated by giving high sugar drinks or food

(d) can be caused by injecting too small a dose of insulin

(e) can be caused by exercise such as gardening or shopping

Ketoacidosis:

(a) may be caused by general illness such as influenza

(b) can be prevented by increasing the insulin dose in accordance with blood glucose testing

(c) can cause sudden unconsciousness without warning

(d) with persistent vomiting will lead to death in 48 h or less if untreated

(e) will always be associated with high urine ketone levels

Microvascular complications in type 1 diabetes:

(a) are not present at the time of diagnosis

(b) are present in almost 100 per cent of people after 25 years of diabetes

(c) affect the lungs and liver mainly

(d) can always be prevented if blood glucose control is good

(e) develop much more slowly if blood pressure is tightly controlled

Chapter 2

Type 2 diabetes:

(a) is partly caused by insulin not working as well as usual

(b) is associated with a steady decline in insulin secretion

(c) occurs rarely in normal weight individuals

(d) tends to be better controlled if regular exercise is taken

(e) is now commonly affecting people under the age of 40 years

Tablet treatment:

(a) metformin can sometimes cause bowel upset

(b) gliclazide stimulates insulin production

(c) gliclazide does not cause hypos

(d) can be expected to work well for decades if the initial response is good

(e) pioglitazone and rosiglitazone are now hardly ever used

Blood glucose:

(a) levels before breakfast are 3.5 – 5.5 mmol/l in people without diabetes

(b) can be tested at home

(c) levels rise after a meal

(d) control can be said to be good if pre-meal readings are over 7 mmol/l

(e) will spill over into urine if levels are over 11 mmol/l

The following are true of complications:

(a) about one third of people with type 2 diabetes will have retinopathy at the time of diagnosis

(b) poor circulation may lead to foot problems

(c) nerve damage may lead to foot problems

(d) good control of blood pressure will decrease the rate of progression of microvascular complications by almost 40 per cent

(e) good control of blood glucose will decrease the rate of progression of microvascular complications by around 25 per cent

Chapter 3

In the eye:

(a) the cornea helps the lens to focus light on the retina

(b) when looking into the distance the lens is pulled into a 'thin' shape

(c) the retina reflects most of the light

(d) the fovea is at the centre of the macula region

(e) the normal ratio of diameters of veins to arteries is 3:2

Background retinopathy:

(a) by itself does not affect vision

(b) includes blot haemorrhages

(c) may indicate the need for tighter blood glucose or blood pressure control

(d) indicates that similar changes may be happening elsewhere in the body

(e) is caused by damage to capillaries of the retina

New vessels:

(a) grow in response to failure of the microcirculation in the retina

(b) arise from the retina, not the optic disc

(c) are fragile and may rupture to release blood

(d) may be present without obvious background change

(e) cause pre-retinal haemorrhage if they rupture

Chapter 4

Blindness:

(a) tends to be a threat earlier in the course of type 2 diabetes compared with type 1 diabetes

(b) is most commonly caused by diabetes at all ages in the UK

(c) is always preceded by several months of visual blurring

(d) has not yet been shown to be reduced by screening programmes

(e) is always caused by proliferative retinopathy whereas maculopathy causes partial sightedness

In a quality assurance programme:

(a) how often the screener reports an image differently to a second expert is measured

(b) a false negative report is one in which the second expert thinks there are abnormalities although the initial report was normal

(c) sensitivity measures how often all abnormals are detected

(d) specificity measures how often normals are reported as abnormal

(e) the recommended sensitivity for detection of sight-threatening retinopathy is over 80 per cent

The following statements are true:

(a) in type 2 diabetes around 20 per cent of people will have proliferative retinopathy after 25 years

(b) in type 2 diabetes around 40 per cent will have exudative maculopathy after 25 years

(c) annual screening is recommended for all people with diabetes

(d) organization of a screening service in a District is the single most important factor in reducing population rates of blindness

(e) laser therapy is effective after visual acuity has decreased in exudative maculopathy

Chapter 5

In the course of retinal screening:

(a) eye appearances are confidential although the diagnosis of diabetes is not

(b) informed consent is necessary before undertaking retinal screening

(c) throughput can be improved by dilating and imaging some people before visual acuity testing

(d) the normal Snellen chart is read at a distance of 6 feet

(e) a pinhole device must always be used.

Visual acuity:

(a) tests retinal function only and the use of usual glasses is not necessary

(b) if the top line cannot be seen, move the subject to 3 m from the chart

(c) a difference of one line (6/18 to 6/24) is significant

(d) can be affected by lighting levels in the room

(e) testing may be impaired by anxiety

Mydriatic drops:

(a) cannot spread infection as they contain a preservative

(b) cause paralysis of accommodation

(c) if tropicamide only is used driving is likely to be safe after 2 h

(d) are always needed to image the retinae of teenagers

(e) must be applied to the cornea to be absorbed

Obtaining the image:

(a) alignment of the split lines is done using the joystick alone

(b) use of the green flashing fixation light is optional for the second and subsequent images

(c) normally the two images of each eye are disc-centred and choroid-centred

(d) image quality must be assessed immediately

(e) eyelashes may cause black lines at the edge of the image

When examining the image:

(a) the disc, vessels and retina are examined in order

(b) a red blur on the disc is not important

(c) variation in colour of the retina is not important

(d) light reflection artefacts are common in older people

(e) the image is not satisfactory unless the arteries are clear after the first branch point

The person with diabetes:

(a) has no right to see their retinal images

(b) waiting for a letter giving results causes no anxiety

(c) is left to take their own diabetes home with them

(d) different words may be necessary to communicate the same information to different people

(e) has more confidence in the retinal screening process if the screener is trained to communicate the results

Classification of appearances:

(a) R1 M0 P1 indicates the need for referral to an ophthalmologist

(b) a blot haemorrhage within one disc diameter of the fovea indicates need for referral to an ophthalmologist

(c) more than 12 blot haemorrhages or microaneurysms must be referred

(d) one pre-retinal haemorrhage must be referred

(e) images which are not clearly interpretable in more than 10 per cent of the area cannot reasonably be reported

Chapters 6–12

Test yourself by opening the book at random, covering the written description and reporting the image. Also, you can access the images on the web at www.servier.co.uk/retinalimagebank and examine them in random order.

Background Information

Driving and diabetes

Anyone holding a driving licence who develops diabetes requiring tablet or insulin therapy must inform the DVLA. This is the patient's responsibility. After starting insulin therapy a patient should not drive until advised that it is safe to do so by their doctor. A medical report will be arranged and normally a 3 year renewable licence will be issued. It is unusual for a driving licence to be withdrawn, but this may happen if a person is taking insulin and becomes unable to detect the early symptoms of hypoglycaemia (as a consequence of long-standing diabetes and over-tight average control). A second reason for the loss of a driving licence is inadequate vision, either because of poor visual acuity or because of poor peripheral vision after laser therapy (note that this is very unusual and only happens when particularly heavy laser therapy has been required to save sight).

People taking insulin cannot hold Heavy Goods Vehicle or Public Service Vehicle licences. Changes to legislation in 2001 allow 'exceptional case' drivers on insulin to hold C1 licences (small lorries).

The 'driving rules' must be followed by all drivers on insulin. They are simple:

(a) test blood glucose before driving;

(b) keep glucose tablets or Lucozade ® in the car;

(c) plan longer journeys to have appropriate stops for snacks and meals.

Handbook of Retinal Screening in Diabetes, Roy Taylor
© 2006 John Wiley & Sons, Ltd

Insurance and diabetes

Everyone must inform their motor insurance company on being diagnosed as having diabetes, however it is treated. Not to do this may invalidate the insurance. The original application form will have specified that the insured must do this.

Unfortunately insurance companies often charge higher premiums for people with diabetes. This is so despite the statistics which show that people with diabetes have less accidents than average. Diabetes UK has negotiated terms with an insurance company, and details can be found on their website (see below).

Employment and diabetes

People with type 2 diabetes should experience little effect on their working life. Exceptions are airline pilots for whom diabetes is a disqualifying condition, and mainline train drivers and Public Service Vehicle licence holders who are barred from these occupations if certain types of tablets (sulphonylureas) are being taken.

For all people requiring insulin therapy there are additional restrictions. Heavy Goods and Public Service Vehicle licences cannot be held. The Police Force, the Fire Service and the Armed services will consider each person individually, and may refuse new employment, whilst transferring those already employed to suitable duties. Deep sea divers are unlikely to be allowed to hold commercial diving licences. Steeplejacks, scaffolders and acrobats need to take extreme care. All driving jobs requiring an ordinary licence or C1 licence should be unaffected apart from restrictions mentioned above in the driving section.

Prescription charges

People with diabetes who are treated with insulin or tablets (but not diet alone) are exempt from prescription charges for medications relating either to diabetes or other conditions. Form AB11 from the general practitioner or Social Security office needs to be completed to obtain the exemption certificate.

British Association of Retinal Screeners (BARS)

This association aims to promote the exchange of practical knowledge and skills between the people who actually carry out retinal screening. It developed from a series of biannual workshops on retinal screening which were held throughout the 1990s. BARS holds annual meetings at which members discuss new information and leaders in screening and related fields are invited to present. More information can be found on the website: http://www. eyescreening.org.uk.

Diabetes UK

The British Diabetic Association was founded in 1934 by the author H.G. Wells and R.D. Lawrence, a doctor who himself had type 1 diabetes. Robin Lawrence developed diabetes in 1920, before insulin was available, and as it was then a fatal condition he went to Florence expecting to die. Early in 1923, when his health was deteriorating badly, he received a telegram: 'Come home. We have insulin.' He went on to found the diabetes clinic at Kings College Hospital, London, and was an inspiration to his patients. His book *The Diabetic Life* laid out the commonsense approach to managing insulin and food which remains valid today. The British Diabetic Association was set up as an organization for patients themselves, to inform and to overcome a general lack of knowledge about diabetes.

In 2002 the name was changed to Diabetes UK. It continues to advise individuals, to publish *Balance*, a bimonthly magazine, to run holidays for young people with diabetes, to support research into diabetes and to organize meetings of all kinds. Local branches exist in many areas, running informative meetings. It is a registered charity (No.215199) and one of its principal activities is to raise money for research and improvements in care.

All people with diabetes are encouraged to join. The contact details are:

Diabetes UK Central Office
10 Parkway, London NW1 7AA
Tel: 020 7424 1000
Fax: 020 7424 1001
Email: info@diabetes.org.uk
Website: http://www.diabetes.org.uk/.

National Retinopathy Screening Systems

The practical information presented in this book should be equally applicable to the slightly different approaches taken in England (http://www.nscretinopathy.org.uk/), Scotland (http://www.nsd.scot.nhs.uk/services/drs/), Wales (http://www.wales.nhs.uk/sites/page.cfm?orgid=351&pid=1903) and Northern Ireland.

Despite slightly different organizational practices in the separate countries, each retinal screener is still dealing with people who need to know about the state of their eyes and their doctors who need to know how retinopathy is changing in order to arrange appropriate management. It is likely that practices will converge to a large degree once the cost effectiveness of different methods has been compared.

Laser therapy

Laser therapy sounds alarming to patients but it is simple and well tolerated. For the patient, it means sitting at a device rather like the screening camera, looking at one place. The ophthalmologist aims the laser beam through the pupil at a precise spot on the retina and administers repeated flashes of laser light. It is not usually painful, and the laser pulses are felt rather as though something was tapping on the eyeball. The eye may ache for a few hours afterwards, and simple analgesics such as paracetamol may be advised. The commonest complaint of patients is that it takes rather a long time and is a tedious procedure. However, it saves sight.

There are two main types of laser therapy.

Pan-retinal photocoagulation is used for proliferative retinopathy. It involves applying several thousand laser dots all over the retina except between the disc and the fovea. Several sessions are usually needed to complete this. Provided that proliferative retinopathy is picked up early enough, pan-retinal photocoagulation is over 95 per cent successful in stopping the process. If vision is preserved after a few months, then the long-term outlook is excellent. For reasons not well understood, once complete treatment has been given and proliferative change has been halted, further new vessel formation is relatively unlikely to reoccur in the future. Naturally, annual retinal screening should be continued.

Grid photocoagulation is used for exudative maculopathy. It involves applying laser spots in a grid pattern lateral to the fovea. It is reasonably successful, but only if visual acuity is better than 6/24 and even then in only about
60 per cent of patients.

The word laser is merely an acronym for the process of producing this
form of light. It stands for *Light Amplification* by the *Stimulated Emission
of Radiation*. Laser light is purely of one wavelength, the waves are all syn-
chronous and the beam is perfectly parallel. It can deliver energy which is
targeted to specific cells or tissues because of these special properties. In treat-
ing diabetic retinopathy, the energy is absorbed by blood in capillaries and
by the pigment epithelium layer.

The only practical problem experienced by people who have required very
heavy laser therapy relates to dim lighting conditions. The pale areas of laser
scar allow internal reflection of light inside the eye with consequent ghost
images. Some visual field defects will be detectable, and formal perimetry is
required to ensure that vision meets the legal requirement to hold a driving
licence.

Vitrectomy

If a large pre-retinal haemorrhage fails to clear, or if fibrous bands threaten to
detach the retina, an operation can be performed to take away the abnormal
tissue. This is done under general anaesthetic. Vitrectomy is performed by
introducing fine instruments through the conjunctiva into the vitreous
humour, with direct vision for the surgeon through the pupil. The abnormal
tissue is cut and sucked out, and clear fluid replaces the volume. If necessary,
laser therapy can be delivered from within the eye. Vision can be dramatically
restored. However, it is a major eye operation and prevention of advanced
changes by effective screening and timely laser therapy is far preferable.

Ophthalmoscopy

Use of the ophthalmoscope can be helpful for retinal screeners, even though
it is not regarded as an essential skill. The ophthalmoscope shines a beam of
light into the eye and allows a view of all the structures from cornea to retina.
It is most useful to sort out what may be preventing a clear view of the retina

(e.g. corneal scarring, cataracts of various sorts and vitreous opacities including asteroid hyalosis). The view is magnified about 15 times, so that some appearances which cannot be assessed fully on the image, even with image manipulation, can be visualized. At first you will be surprised that you can only see an area about the size of the disc at any one time, and you have to move this 'searchlight' back and forth across the retina to build up a full picture. It is a difficult skill, but once obtained makes screening easier and more interesting.

1. *Getting started.* Hold the ophthalmoscope in your right hand (this is easier to start for right handers). Switch on the light (usually by rotating a collar) and check that the lens is set to zero by rotating the focus wheel, going through the circle of convex and concave lenses at the head of the scope. Rest the top of the instrument firmly in the angle between your right eyebrow and nose so that (with some jiggling) you can see through the viewing hole. Look around the room. Find the light switch. You should get used to moving your head and the scope as a single unit.

2. *Look in an eye.* With your subject sitting comfortably and you standing in front, decide where to ask him/her to look. This should be at a distinct point, not in the middle of a blank wall. It should be in a position so that your subject's line of gaze passes the level of your eyes (usually at about 60° elevation). Place your left hand on your subject's forehead with your thumb along the right eyebrow. Close your left eye. Starting at arm's length, look through the scope at the right pupil. Move slowly towards the eye. You should see redness when 30–50 cm from the eye. Closer up, everything will appear pink and blurred. You can confidently move to within 2.5 cm of the eye as your forehead will make contact with your left thumb safely before the scope gets too close to the eye. Look around. You may see a blood vessel or two.

3. *Relax.* Go back to looking round the room through the scope. This time place your right forefinger on the focus wheel and click it round, one step at a time. Your view will get fuzzier, then change suddenly as the lens gets to the point of the strongest + correction next to the strongest – correction. Get used to focusing without moving the scope.

4. *Now you have learned the basic moves* you can start on the clinically useful systematic approach. Repeat step 2, but ensure that you move towards

the eye along a line about 15° to the side of the line of gaze. This will mean that you are lined up on the optic disc. Ask yourself these questions: (a) cornea OK?; (b) lens clear?; (c) vitreous clear? If you encounter no abnormalities you should be looking at the retina at or near the optic disc. Pivot your line of sight through your subject's pupil. When you can see a blood vessel, turn the focus wheel one way then the other to get the sharpest possible view. Next, follow that blood vessel one way then the other until you come to the optic disc.

5. *And then the other eye.* For right handers, using the left eye and the left hand is more awkward at first. All the above instructions should be left–right reversed. You will stand in front and just to the left of your subject, looking into his / her left eye with your left eye, holding the scope with your left hand. Ophthalmoscopy is not easy, and needs months of practice before you can expect to be confident.

6. *Common problems crop up* such as: I cannot close one eye, I wear glasses, I can't focus. The brief answers are: cover it with a hand rather than resting it on the forehead, take them off, practice focusing on your hand from about 10 cm away. Ask an expert to help with your ophthalmoscopy.

Answers to Self-assessment Questions

Chapter 1

Type 1 diabetes:

(a) No – failure of the beta cells

(b) Yes

(c) No – there is some tendency but only type 2 has a strong tendency to run in families

(d) Yes

(e) Yes

At the time of diagnosis of type 1 diabetes:

(a) Yes

(b) No – symptoms tend to have come on recently

(c) No – thrush and boils are both fairly common and may be the reason that a person consults their doctor

(d) Yes

(e) Yes

Handbook of Retinal Screening in Diabetes, Roy Taylor
© 2006 John Wiley & Sons, Ltd

For treatment of type 1 diabetes, insulin:

(a) No – into the fat layer

(b) Yes

(c) Yes

(d) Yes

(e) Yes

Eating in type 1 diabetes:

(a) No – around carbohydrate counting and low fat content

(b) No – by estimating the carbohydrate content

(c) Yes

(d) No – a small potato is one 10 g portion

(e) Yes

Hypoglycaemia:

(a) Yes

(b) No – hypoglycaemic unawareness is dangerous if present

(c) Yes

(d) No – too large a dose of insulin

(e) Yes

Ketoacidosis:

(a) Yes

(b) Yes

(c) No – it is always preceded by some degree of illness

(d) Yes

(e) Yes

Microvascular complications in type 1 diabetes:

(a) Yes

(b) Yes

(c) No – retinas, nerves and kidney

(d) No – the susceptibility to complications varies

(e) Yes

Chapter 2

Type 2 diabetes:

(a) Yes

(b) Yes

(c) Yes

(d) Yes

(e) Yes

Tablet treatment:

(a) Yes

(b) Yes

(c) No – gliclazide can cause hypos

(d) No – the ability to produce insulin gradually decreases and control worsens

(e) No – pioglitazone and rosiglitazone are new insulin sensitizers

Blood glucose:

(a) Yes

(b) Yes

(c) Yes

(d) No – good if pre-meal readings are under 7 mmol/l

(e) Yes

The following are true of complications:

(a) Yes

(b) Yes

(c) Yes

(d) Yes

(e) Yes

Chapter 3

In the eye:

(a) Yes

(b) Yes

(c) No – the retina lets the light through and the black choroid absorbs it

(d) Yes

(e) Yes

Background retinopathy:

(a) Yes

(b) Yes

(c) Yes

(d) Yes

(e) Yes

New vessels:

(a) Yes

(b) No – from either the retina or the optic disc

(c) Yes

(d) Yes

(e) Yes

Chapter 4

Blindness:

(a) Yes

(b) No – only in the working age population (macula degeneration is commonest in the elderly and overall in the UK)

(c) No – it may be sudden in proliferative disease

(d) No – reduced by screening programmes in both Sweden and Newcastle

(e) No – maculopathy is the more common cause of blindness

In a quality assurance programme:

(a) Yes

(b) Yes

(c) Yes

(d) Yes

(e) Yes

The following statements are true:

(a) Yes

(b) No – around 20 per cent will have exudative maculopathy after 25 years

(c) Yes

(d) Yes

(e) No – laser therapy will not restore vision in exudative maculopathy

Chapter 5

In the course of retinal screening:

(a) No – all information is confidential

(b) Yes

(c) No – visual acuity must be tested before mydriasis

(d) No – 6 metres

(e) No – a pinhole device is used when glasses are not available or if VA appears low

Visual acuity:

(a) No – refraction, the clarity of lens/vitreous and retinal function are tested

(b) Yes

(c) No – only a two line difference is significant

(d) Yes

(e) Yes

Mydriatic drops:

(a) No – full precautions must always be taken

(b) Yes

(c) Yes

(d) No – young people can be sometimes imaged satisfactorily without mydriasis but time must be left between image acquisitions for the pupil to re-dilate

(e) No – they are rapidly spread across the conjunctiva and cornea by blinking

Obtaining the image:

(a) No – joystick first then fine focusing knob

(b) No – essential for all images

(c) No – disc-centred and macula-centred

(d) Yes

(e) No – pale streaks at the edge of the image

When examining the image:

(a) Yes

(b) No – a red blur on the disc may indicate new vessels – examine closely

(c) Yes

(d) No – common in younger people

(e) No – after the second branch points

The person with diabetes:

(a) No – the image is theirs

(b) No – waiting for results can be a cause of anxiety

(c) Yes

(d) Yes

(e) Yes

Classification of appearances:

(a) No – background with previous laser

(b) No – two blot haemorrhages within one disc diameter from the fovea together with a VA of less than 6/12 indicates need for referral on current criteria

(c) No – simple background retinopathy should not be referred

(d) Yes

(e) No – more than 25 per cent of the area not clear is unacceptable

Glossary of Terms

Aqueous humour. The watery fluid which fills the space behind the cornea and in front of the lens (the anterior chamber).

Arteriole. The smallest branches of arteries supplying tissue. In this book the word 'artery' is used for simplicity to cover both arteriole and artery.

Artery. Blood vessel carrying oxygenated blood from the heart under pressure.

AV nipping. This refers to the optical illusion of a vein being squeezed by an artery crossing over. As there is no physical nipping, it is often referred to as 'AV crossing change'. It indicates high blood pressure.

Beta cells. The beta cells of the islets within the pancreas produce insulin. The islets also contain other kinds of hormone producing cells.

Capillary. The smallest blood vessel, which has a lining only one cell thick.

Carbohydrate. The component of food which can be broken down by the body into glucose. Carbohydrate intake is estimated as 10 g exchanges (e.g. one small potato is a 10 g exchange).

Choroid. The black lining to the eyeball which prevents reflection of light.

Ciliary muscle. The circular muscle which contracts to allow the lens to become thickened, allowing focusing on very near objects.

Circinate. This refers to the occurrence of exudates which appear to be arranged on the circumference of a circle. The circle does not necessarily need to be complete. There is likely to be a leaky blood vessel at the centre of the circle.

Handbook of Retinal Screening in Diabetes, Roy Taylor
© 2006 John Wiley & Sons, Ltd

Clinically significant macula oedema. This can only be diagnosed using binocular vision and a slit lamp, and consists of thickening of the retina close to the fovea caused by fluid swelling.

Cones. The light detector cells which can detect colour and are concentrated in the fovea.

Conjunctiva. The white covering of the eye which is visible on inspecting the external eye.

Diabetes. A long-term condition characterized by high levels of glucose (sugar) in the blood.

Fovea. The centre of the macular region where all detailed vision is registered.

Glucagon. The hormone which has the opposite effect to that of insulin and causes the liver to produce glucose. It is part of the body's normal control mechanisms, and is also used as an injectable medicine to treat severe hypoglycaemia.

Glucose. The form of sugar to which all carbohydrate food is broken down in the body. The concentration of glucose in the blood is normally very tightly controlled.

HbA1c. This is the percentage of red blood cell pigment (haemoglobin) which has become attached to glucose. It is used as an indicator of the average blood glucose over the previous 8 weeks.

Hypoglycaemia. Hypo means low, and glycaemia refers to blood glucose. The word is usually shortened to 'hypo'.

Insulin. The hormone produced by the beta cells in the pancreas which acts to decrease blood glucose (sugar) levels.

Iris. The coloured part of the eye which regulates the amount of light permitted to enter.

IRMA. This stands for intra retinal microvascular anomaly and refers to small vessels which have become very dilated and appear then disappear on the retina not obviously connected to larger vessels.

Ketoacidosis. A potentially fatal condition which occurs when a person with type 1 diabetes has not taken enough insulin for the circumstances (e.g. other illness), and there are high levels of ketones and glucose in the blood and urine.

Ketones. The by-product of fat breakdown, and trace amounts can be found in the urine of anyone during fasting. Very large amounts of ketones in the urine suggest that there is not enough insulin to prevent excessive fat breakdown.

Logmar chart. A chart for measuring visual acuity which differentiates more satisfactorily between degrees of severe visual impairment and is therefore used by ophthalmologists rather than population screening services.

Macrovascular. This term applies to deposition of fat in the walls of arteries increasing the risk of heart attack and stroke and reducing circulation to the feet.

Macula. The area between the upper and lower arcades of vessels, bounded by the optic disc nasally and two disc diameter from the fovea on the temporal side.

Maculopathy. This term refers to disease within one disc diameter of the fovea. It may be exudative, cystoid or ischaemic and may be associated with 'clinically significant macula oedema'.

Microvascular. This term refers to complications caused by the damage to capillaries in the retina, nerves and kidney.

Mydriasis. The process of dilating the pupil using eye drops, usually tropicamide in screening programmes.

Myelinated. This refers to the sheath which surrounds nerve fibres in many parts of the body, but not usually in the retina.

Nasal. The side of a retinal image nearest the nose. The optic disc is always nasal to the fovea.

Oedema. This refers to the presence of excess fluid in a tissue.

Ophthalmoscope. An instrument with a light source and a series of lenses to allow direct inspection of the retina. The technique requires considerable expertise.

Optic disc. The pale rounded area of the retina where nerve fibres gather together to form the head of the optic nerve.

Oral hypoglycaemic agent. This term refers to tablets used in type 2 diabetes to control blood glucose.

Pancreas. The organ which lies behind the stomach and has two functions. First, digestive juices are passed directly into the intestine. Secondly, clusters of hormone producing cells called islets pass insulin and other hormones into the blood stream.

Papilloedema. This is swelling of the head of the optic nerve which causes the disc to be pink, the disc margins to be blurred and the veins to be very dilated.

Pen injector. A device which holds a cartridge of insulin and can be used to administer an insulin injection without having to draw up insulin into a syringe from a vial.

Proliferative retinopathy. This refers to the growth of fragile new vessels which are at risk of bleeding and causing loss of vision.

Refraction. When a ray of light passes from one substance to another of a different density (e.g. air/glass or air/cornea) the ray of light changes direction. Rays of light entering the eye are refracted first at the corneal surface and then at the lens to be focused on the retina.

Retina. The light-sensitive tissue at the back of the eye.

Retinal screener. A member of the Diabetes Care Team characterized by empathy with patients, knowledge and skill in retinal screening and outstanding ability to communicate with the patient, doctor and ophthalmologist.

Rods. Light detector cells which only detect the presence of light, not its colour, but which are sensitive to low light levels. They provide all peripheral vision (i.e. everywhere around the point of gaze).

Snellen chart. The standard chart for testing visual acuity.

Sclera. The tough white layer which forms the outer covering of the eyeball.

Sensitivity. A measure of how complete the screening process is in detecting all positive findings.

Specificity. A term used in quality assurance to indicate how good the system is in avoiding indication of a positive finding when in fact this is not so.

Suspensory ligaments. The elastic structure which tends to pull the lens into a thin shape unless the circular ciliary muscle is contracting.

Temporal. This term refers to the side of a retinal image closest to the side of the head (the temple).

Vein. Blood vessel carrying blood from the tissues back towards the heart.

Vitreous humour. The dense jelly-like substance filling the globe of the eye.

Index

Note: Figures and Tables are indicated by *italic page numbers*